Under the Mask

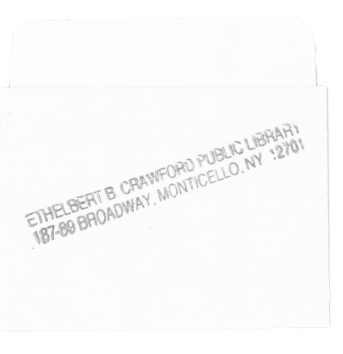

Under the Mask

· · ·

A Guide to Feeling Secure and Comfortable during Anesthesia and Surgery

· · ·

James E. Cottrell, M.D.
with Stephanie Golden

· · ·

Illustrations by Tay McClellan

RUTGERS UNIVERSITY PRESS
New Brunswick, New Jersey, and London

Library of Congress Cataloging-in-Publication Data

Cottrell, James E.

Under the mask : a guide to feeling secure and comfortable during anesthesia
and surgery / James E. Cottrell with Stephanie Golden.

p.   cm.

Includes bibliographical references and index.

ISBN 0–8135–2877–1 (cloth : alk. paper) — ISBN 0–8135–2878–X (paper :
alk. paper)

1. Anesthesiology—Popular works.   2. Anesthesia—Popular works.
3. Managed care plans (Medical care)   4. Consumer education.   I. Golden,
Stephanie.   II. Title.

RD81 .C72 2001
617.9′6—dc21   00-034202

British Cataloging-in-Publication data for this book is available from the
British Library.

Manufactured in the United States of America

This book is dedicated to the memory of Diane Cleaver,
a friend and agent who encouraged its writing; her enthusiasm
fueled my desire to complete it.

This book is also dedicated to all the doctors who have made
the specialty of anesthesiology so safe for everyone having surgery.
They have made such progress in conquering all types of pain
that, as time goes on, fewer and fewer people will feel
a need for assisted suicide.

Contents

• • •

CONTENTS

Acknowledgments

• • •

First, I acknowledge Stephanie Golden for her intelligence, dedication, and hard work in preparing this important book. She enabled my voice to be heard, and luckily hers is present as well.

I thank all those who reviewed chapters: Audrée Bendo, Neal Cohen, Paul Dadic, Christophe DeBrady, Timothy Deer, Carl Fischer, David Fishman, George Gabrielson, Adrian Gelb, Alexander Gotta, Paul Grube, Roberta Hines, Samuel Hughes, Banu Lokhandwala, Vinod Malholtra, Catherine McWade, Michael Mulroy, Mark Rosen, René Templehoff, Richard Traysman, Rebecca Twersky, David Wlody, and Dan Zabel; as well as Warren Zapol, Joseph Lovett, Maribeth Winslow, and John Hoffman.

I thank Helen Hsu for her support and encouragement from the very beginning of this project, as well as for her perceptive help in shaping the text. I am also grateful to Willow Krienke who did the copyediting, Brigitte Goldstein and the rest of the staff of Rutgers University Press for their high level of professionalism, which has enhanced this book's potential contribution to the well being of medical consumers across the country.

I thank those who shared stories with me: Deborah Kass, Alice Sachs Zimet, Stacey Harris, Margaret Kern, and especially Robert Lipsyte, who always has time to read and comment on my writings. Thanks also to John Hartung, who has encouraged and helped develop my writing and speaking skills over the years. Thanks to Medtronic for advice on implantable devices.

Finally, I thank Anne Minaidis, my perfect assistant.

Under the Mask

PART 1

• • •

Basic Information

• • •

CHAPTER 1

• • •

Introduction:
Anesthesiology's New Role

• • •

Some years ago, while waiting outside my office as medical students arrived for an introduction to anesthesiology, I overheard one ask a fellow student, "What is anesthesiology?" The response: "Putting people to sleep."

I walked in, introduced myself, and asked them to imagine the following:

"You're lying face up on a table, covered by a sheet. A surgeon comes up, pulls the sheet off, and makes an incision in your skin over your breastbone. He then cuts through your breastbone and spreads your chest apart so he can reach your heart.

"Hooking your blood circulation up to a pump, he removes a valve from your heart and replaces it with a valve from a pig. Finally he restores the blood flow through your heart, puts it back in place, and closes up your chest.

"How many of you could sleep through that?"

They laughed and fidgeted, realizing that I had overheard the student's question. But they got my point. It's much easier to say that anesthesiologists "put people to sleep" than to explain the complexity of what they actually do.

An anesthesiologist disarms the entire nervous system with the most powerful drugs known to medicine; keeps you alive while you're subjected to manipulations that would otherwise kill you; and finally miraculously reanimates you. Truly, the superficial analogy between anesthesia and sleep hardly does justice to this phenomenal medical intervention, which is exciting, wonderful, and still more mysterious than understood.

All too long, we've been the unseen doctors. But in fact, the anesthesiologist is one of the most important physicians you'll encounter during your experience of surgery. He or she is your caretaker while the surgeon is busy cutting and stitching. Most people don't realize the significance of the anesthesiologist's contribution both to their safety and comfort during surgery and recovery and to their ultimate well-being.

For example, anesthesia can have lasting psychological effects. Dr. Aaron Beck, the founder of cognitive therapy, told the *New York Times* how an experience with anesthesia at age eight shaped his entire life. After surgery for a broken arm, he remembered the surgeon saying, "He's not under yet," then recalled a "terrible dream" of a string of alligators, each biting the next one's tail, with the last one biting his arm. He also recalled his mother repeating, "He will not die."

This experience left the young Aaron Beck with "a phobia of blood and injury." In reaction to a hospital scene in a movie, his blood pressure would drop (in some people, anxiety stimulates the parasympathetic nervous system, which by relaxing the blood vessels causes low blood pressure). What was more, the scent of ether made him faint (Sally, whose story begins chapter 17, had a very similar reaction). In a foreshadowing of his cognitive approach to psychotherapy, Beck finally overcame these irrational fears through the use of logic.

In the past twenty years, anesthesia has expanded far beyond its role in the operating room. Today it is an extremely complex specialty that has branched into a number of subspecialties, such as obstetrics, neurosurgery, and pain control. During this same period, the increasing dominance of managed care has radically changed the environment in which health care is provided. One effect of these developments is that you, the medical consumer, need to know more than did patients in the past about what anesthesiologists do, not only to get the best of what they have to offer but to protect your well-being.

Over the years we've decreased the risk of injury in anesthesia to the point where it's now quite safe. In the vast majority of cases, having anesthesia is like having a baby—everything goes well and you come out of it feeling fine. But there remains a low risk of serious injury or even death; one fatality occurs for every 250,000 times anesthesia is given.

Some years ago the TV program "Day One" highlighted this risk in reporting a case in which having a baby did not turn out well. The anesthesiologist for a woman having a cesarean section had to leave the operating room to care for another patient, and no competent replacement was provided. During his absence the mother's oxygen supply became too low, and she emerged from the birth brain-damaged, unable to care properly for her child.

Yet this calamity could have been averted. As I'll explain more fully in chapter 4, patients can take steps to ensure that the anesthesiologist remains in the operating room or is readily available throughout the procedure. In the current health care environment, where the time physicians have to spend with patients is sharply limited, it is increasingly up to the patient to become an informed consumer and take charge. I've written *Under the Mask* to empower you with the knowledge you need to do this.

To bolster your knowledge of your rights as a patient, I'll discuss the new, expanded roles of anesthesiology within the context of managed care. For all the different conditions covered in this book, I'll tell you what to expect, what to do if you feel you're not getting what you need, and—depending on the seriousness of your condition—how far you should be willing to go to get it. Once the surgical process is demystified and you know how to get the best possible care, you'll feel more comfortable and less stressed when facing surgery, which itself is a significant factor improving outcome.

Empowering You to Protect Yourself: Two Principles

I really hate going down to the preadmission testing unit in our hospital because it's always filled with people sitting there saying, "I don't want to know anything about the anesthesia—just put me out!" They're simply refusing any responsibility for decisions about managing their own care. What I'd like to see instead is patients who know the options that are available to them, both for anesthesia during surgery and for pain control afterward, and take an active part in deciding what's best for them.

Each year about 40 million Americans require surgery. In my many years as an anesthesiologist, I've learned that most people don't understand what's going to happen to them during medical procedures. Because they feel helpless, unable to protect themselves, they simply put their trust in the doctor. Today, however, you need to protect yourself by acquiring some basic knowledge about anesthesiology and about how the health care system functions.

There are two basic principles of being an informed medical consumer:

- Give the anesthesiologist all the information needed to protect you.
- Know how to ask questions—about the procedures that will be used, and about anything else that concerns you.

Under the Mask provides the detailed information you need to act on these principles for all the most common surgical procedures performed today. This knowledge will put you in control—able to make choices that shape your care.

Provide the Right Information

This first principle is critical because, under managed care, your anesthesiologist may not have the time to sit you down and ask probing questions about your condition; in fact, you may not see the anesthesiologist before surgery at all. It's up to you to provide a complete medical history—including details that may seem trivial. A few examples will illustrate the importance of this information.

During an emergency preoperative consultation with a patient scheduled for a hernia repair, the anesthesiologist's examination revealed numerous bruises under the skin. Questioning the patient, she found that he was taking aspirin regularly two or three times a day—something he had failed to disclose. (Aspirin interferes with blood coagulation, causing bleeding under the skin just from minor bumps.) She therefore changed her anesthetic plan, deciding to give him general instead of regional anesthesia. Making this change avoided the remote possibility that a hematoma (collection of blood) might form around the patient's spine and cause weakness or paraplegia (paralysis) of the legs. That would have required additional surgery to drain the hematoma.

In another case, a friend of mine who had had a heart attack underwent an angioplasty (a procedure to dilate a narrowed coronary artery). During the procedure the artery being dilated ruptured, necessitating emergency cardiac surgery. The anesthesiologist suddenly called to transport the patient to the operating room had, of course, never seen him before. Since there was no history in the chart regarding previous anesthetics, he used a standard anesthetic. The patient immediately turned red and developed hives, asthma (contraction of the air passages of the lungs, constricting breathing), and hypotension (low blood pressure). Recognizing this as a life-threatening allergic reaction, the anesthesiologist was able to treat it, and the patient survived. After the surgery the patient told the anesthesiologist that he knew he was allergic to that standard anesthetic drug.

In still another case, a young woman having a hysterectomy did not have a preoperative consultation. Instead she was given a printed checklist to fill out, which asked for details of her medical history: medications taken, allergies, previous surgery, and so on. Because her English was poor, she did not fully complete the form.

During the operation, after inducing anesthesia, the anesthesiologist began the routine practice of inserting an endotracheal tube (which goes down the windpipe) to enable the patient to breathe, and only then discovered that the tube could not be placed because of an anatomical deformity in her jaw. Had he known about this in advance, he could have been better prepared to deal with it. Luckily, he was skilled enough to provide the anesthesia safely without the tube. After the operation, using an interpreter, the anesthesiologist learned that she had had the same problem in a previous operation. If she had had a preoperative consultation with an interpreter present, this near emergency could have been avoided.

An elderly woman came to our preoperative clinic for evaluation before cataract surgery. The anesthesiologist discovered that she had very high blood pressure (170/110) and told her to see her primary care doctor to reduce it. When he saw her again two weeks later, her blood pressure was still too high (160/100). Questioned, she explained that the primary care doctor had not had time to see her and had called in a prescription to her pharmacist. The prescription was for a diuretic, the standard drug given initially to lower blood pressure. In this case, the diuretic was not potent enough, and the physician had not done a follow-up to see whether it was effective. The anesthesiologist called the primary care doctor to inform him that the patient required a more potent drug. Two weeks later she returned with her blood pressure adequately lowered, and the cataract was removed safely.

In all these cases, a skilled practitioner was able to cope with an unexpected problem and avert a possible complication. But it would have been much safer had the patients been aware in the first place of what the anesthesiologist needed to know in order to perform the procedure safely.

Know How to Ask Questions

The second principle of being an informed consumer involves knowing what questions to ask and how to ask them. For example, the mother who was injured during her cesarean section could have protected herself by asking:

- Who will be doing my anesthesia?
- Will that person be present throughout the procedure?
- Who will be assisting, and will the assistant be left in charge at any point? If so, will the anesthesiologist be in the hospital, readily available within a few minutes?

Asking the right questions also means not letting yourself be deterred by discomfort or embarrassment. Recently a woman was referred to our hospital for specialized surgery on her neck and the base of her skull. She came with all her paperwork and was seen by an anesthesiologist the day before surgery. The next morning, as the intravenous, arterial, and central venous pressure lines (catheters used for monitoring and maintaining blood pressure) were being placed, the operative team noticed continued bleeding at the sites where the catheters were inserted. They quickly administered a standard test for duration of bleeding after a puncture. The result was grossly abnormal, and the surgery was canceled, even though all the invasive monitors had already been inserted.

When the patient awakened, she admitted she had been taking high doses of ibuprofen, which, like aspirin, interferes with blood coagulation. She confessed that she had wanted to ask whether this would affect her surgery, but had been reluctant to do so because she hesitated to reveal that she used so much of it. And since it was an over-the-counter drug, she finally decided that she didn't have to mention it.

The message here is: Ask the question, no matter how unimportant you think it may be, and even if you fear embarrassment. Your doctors will not be shocked—they've heard everyone's secrets, and they're there to help.

There is one other important aspect of this second principle of knowing what to ask:

- Know what procedures are available and appropriate for different types of surgery or diagnostic procedures, so you can ask for them if they haven't been offered.

Once you've read this book you'll be aware of all the anesthetic procedures that are available to make you safer and more comfortable, even if your doctor hasn't suggested them. If you ask for them, often you can get them.

Anesthesiology's New Roles

In the past, anesthesiologists focused on pain relief during surgery. They were seldom seen outside the operating room—whether in the hospital, a freestanding ambulatory surgery center, or a surgeon's office. Today, we spend half our time outside the operating room, mostly in our offices seeing patients like other doctors.

- We see many patients before their surgery in order to assess their medical history and condition. We plan with them the type of surgical anesthetic to be used and decide together what kind of postoperative pain relief will be best for them.

- Our second most important role outside the operating room is assisting with radiological diagnostic procedures such as MRIs, CAT scans, and angiograms, as well as with all types of procedures involving endoscopes (instruments allowing visualization of the interior of a hollow organ). These procedures might include biopsies of the lungs and trachea (windpipe) and polyp removal from the colon.
- Our third role is pain management for acute postoperative pain and for chronic pain.
- In our fourth role, we care for patients in the critical care unit who may be in shock, suffering respiratory failure, or experiencing complications resulting from surgery or trauma.

In 1969, when I began my residency, there were approximately ten thousand anesthesiologists in the United States. Today, nearly thirty-eight thousand physicians limit their practice to this specialty, and over 65 percent of them spend a great deal of their time in a subspecialty.

The development of the anesthetic subspecialties grew out of a recognition that different groups of people have widely varying reactions to anesthetics and thus need different care. For example, in obstetrics the effects of anesthetics are unique by comparison to other areas of anesthesia. In addition, the two lives involved are completely different from each other physiologically and thus respond differently to anesthetics.

The anesthetic subspecialties are pediatrics, obstetrics, neurosurgery, cardiac surgery, critical care, pain management, transplant surgery, trauma surgery, and ambulatory surgery. A physician who is "board certified" in anesthesia has satisfied the requirements of the American Board of Anesthesiology. The board gives a written exam at the end of a three-year training period to assess the physician's knowledge. The physician must then take an oral exam, involving discussions of clinical case management, to assess competence.

A "board-eligible" physician is working his or her way through this system in order to become certified. The doctor has several chances to take the written and oral exams; becoming board certified can take as long as six years. It would be optimal to be cared for by a specialist when your medical problem falls into one of the subspecialty categories, but even if a specialist is not available, an anesthesiologist who has some expertise in that area can certainly perform the procedure safely.

For example, our hospital recently received certification from the state to perform liver transplants. We recruited an anesthesiologist who had done a year's fellowship in liver transplant anesthesia. Since we anticipated doing only five transplants the first year, we felt that he could manage all five. However, he was unable to perform the fourth one, since his wife had just gone into labor.

A few phone calls located another anesthesiologist on the staff who had participated in about twenty-five liver transplants during his residency. With his previous experience, the use of a protocol written by the specialist who was away, and the help of the experienced surgeon, the transplant was performed successfully, avoiding the need to transfer the patient to another hospital.

The Anesthesiologist at Work

There is considerable truth in the common perception that you face a greater risk from anesthesia than from surgery itself. Rapid changes in your medical status occur during surgery. There can be blood loss, shifts in blood pressure, changes in heart rate and rhythm, decreases in urine output, and sudden breathing difficulties. As you'll see in chapter 3, where I give a blow-by-blow description of the anesthesiologist's role in the operating room, all these reactions require swift, on-the-spot responses. The anesthesiologist must place and read monitors to detect changes in the patient's status, administer fluids and drugs to correct them, and interpret the monitors to evaluate the effectiveness of these measures.

The physiological and pharmacological knowledge required, plus the skills needed to place and interpret the monitors, make the anesthesiologist's job quite different from the surgeon's. Surgery is a technical skill; the surgeon must know what to cut and how. The anesthesiologist's job is to maintain life while the surgeon does this, so he or she is concerned with the patient's medical condition as a whole.

Jerry came to the hospital for repair of an inguinal hernia. About a week earlier he had seen his anesthesiologist, who learned of numerous medical problems that he was being treated for. He had chronic obstructive pulmonary disease due to heavy smoking, including a chronic cough and bronchitis. He also had high blood pressure, for which he had been given medication.

Since both these conditions had to be brought under control before the surgery, the anesthesiologist stressed the importance of taking his medication as prescribed—which Jerry hadn't been doing. She also recommended that his primary care doctor add another medication, an antibiotic, to treat the bronchitis and prevent pneumonia from developing after the operation.

Jerry had his surgery under a regional anesthetic, chosen because it would interfere least with his lung disease and high blood pressure. During the procedure, however, his blood pressure suddenly dropped; his speech slurred, and he became confused. The anesthesiologist promptly raised his blood pressure by administering a vasopressor (a drug that stimulates contraction of the blood vessels), and the symptoms disappeared.

Upon questioning, Jerry said he'd had these symptoms before but hadn't thought they were important enough to mention. This answer alerted the anesthesiologist to watch him closely postoperatively, since his symptoms during surgery signaled that he'd been having a transient ischemic attack, which indicates disease of the carotid arteries (which supply blood to the brain). She also referred him to a neurologist, who did further testing that eventually led to carotid artery surgery.

Jerry's case illustrates the global nature of the anesthesiologist's role. Not only was his anesthesiologist able to treat him during surgery, prevent him from having a stroke in the operating room, she also identified a serious disease he had and wasn't aware of, enabling him to get treatment before the disease itself caused a stroke.

You Don't Have to Be in Pain

Under the Mask will bring you up to date on the great advances that have occurred recently in our ability to ease pain of all kinds. In the past, as we will see in chapter 2, physicians had very few ways to control pain. They developed the attitude that patients' complaints of pain were to be ignored. This state of mind prevailed for centuries and is still widespread today, despite the development of new techniques that enable us to relieve pain more effectively than ever before.

In obstetrics, the old attitude was reinforced by the ancient notion that it is women's role to suffer in giving birth, a belief that derives from God's curse on Eve ("in pain you shall bring forth children"). In the nineteenth century, when methods of pain relief were unsafe and mothers who had anesthesia during childbirth were often harmed by it, such an attitude might have had practical value. But today it has no medical justification.

There also remains a reluctance to fully relieve other types of pain, which is reinforced by the derogatory connotations of drug addiction. Society's abhorrence of drug addicts has tainted the idea that narcotics should be used to control chronic pain, such as from cancer. This old-fashioned prejudice is still alive and well, even among physicians.

Helen had severe, incapacitating pain due to breast cancer that had metastasized to her bones, including her skull. Her primary care doctor referred her to an anesthesiologist who was a pain specialist. He gave her a low-dose form of morphine that she would have to take for the rest of her life, since the pain would continue to increase. When the primary care doctor learned of this, he was outraged. He called the pain specialist and demanded, "What are you trying to do—make my patient an addict?" He took for granted that it was inappropriate to give Helen narcotics, even though her pain would only worsen until the cancer killed her.

This doctor's response represented a spillover of the common attitude toward addicts to someone who had a real need for pain-relieving medications. For physiological reasons that I'll explain in chapter 16, people with this real need usually don't become addicted when given narcotics. Today there's absolutely no reason for most people to have pain because there are so many options for relieving it. These new methods of pain relief are generally without harmful side effects, since we now have different ways of administering drugs like morphine, which did have adverse effects with the older methods.

As a result, most people can die without pain even from the worst cancers, such as pancreatic or metastatic breast cancer. Many people with debilitating conditions, such as low back pain, can return to their jobs. I've seen people who hadn't worked for five years come to a pain specialist and within months go back to work and lead a productive, normal life. Yet many sufferers aren't aware of this and assume they have to live with their pain.

In the following chapters, I recommend narcotics for relief of postoperative pain or to allay preoperative stress. You can ask your anesthesiologist for these drugs and be confident that you are not being weak or soft or courting a dangerous dependency.

How to Use This Book

Under the Mask will take you through all of the most common surgical procedures performed today, as well as pain control techniques for both postoperative and chronic pain. Part 1 presents the basic information you will need to understand anesthesiology's new roles in medical care. It describes the development and current scope of anesthesiology, the medications and techniques we use, and our various roles inside and outside the operating room. It explains your rights as a patient and tells you how to use whatever time is available to consult with your anesthesiologist to best effect, specifying what information to provide and what questions to ask.

Finally, part 1 describes the constraints on anesthesiologists within the structure of managed care and explains how you can often work with your doctor to expand the options available to you. Many physicians would be delighted to have patients demand care that their HMO refuses on the basis of cost.

I suggest you read through all five chapters in part 1, since they contain information you'll need to understand much of the medical material in part 2. You can then turn to the specific chapter in part 2 that covers your particular medical concern. I explain what each procedure is like, what issues it raises for anesthesia, what the particular risks may be, and what specific questions to ask the anesthesiologist.

Why I Became an Anesthesiologist

My interest in relieving pain grows out of a series of experiences during my youth that seared the devastating effects of pain into my awareness, paving my own path toward becoming an anesthesiologist. As a nine-year-old, I watched in horror as my father lay dying from metastatic cancer. I didn't understand the concept of dying, although my mother tried to explain it to me and my sister. I did understand the agony on my father's face as the cancer ate away at his spine. At that time, the only available form of pain relief was injection of morphine into a muscle. Not only was this method of administering morphine ineffective for my father, its side effects of nausea, disorientation, constipation, and dry mouth only added to his discomfort. His pain was so severe that increasing the morphine enough to relieve it would have stopped his breathing.

Today, however, we have several techniques that could have relieved my father's pain: nerve blocks using local anesthetics, continuous infusion around the spinal cord of a combination of narcotics and local anesthetics, or permanent nerve ablations (which destroy nerve tissue).

Shortly before my father died, I stepped on broken glass, and our family doctor decided that it had to be surgically removed. He froze the bottom of my foot with ethyl chloride, a local anesthetic, not once but many times as he hunted for the tiny shards like so many needles in a haystack. The ethyl chloride was ineffective, and the pain was unbearable, soothed only by my mother's quiet songs.

As a result of these and other experiences, I decided to become a doctor. When I learned in medical school about the specialty of anesthesiology, I could look back and see where I would have been of great assistance—to my father, to a boy like myself during the operation on my foot, or to the young polio victims I had assisted in a local hospital after an epidemic, who required life support and extensive rehabilitation.

One of my first patients in medical school was a thirty-four-year-old woman with leukemia who needed intensive care and constant supervision during the last few months of her life. I saw how our care enabled her children to visit, which was critically important for them. Later, as a third-year student, I was assisting in the operating room when the patient on the table went into cardiac arrest. The anesthesiologist took charge and revived the patient. I was impressed. I thought, "Who is that guy?"

In this way I became aware of the tremendous value to society of relieving pain and prolonging life. At the time there were very few doctors who specialized in anesthesia, but over the past twenty-five years I've seen great changes. I've written this book to share my knowledge so that other people can take more advantage of the opportunities offered by this remarkable specialty—because we don't just "put people to sleep."

Summary: Questions and Points to Remember

- Give the anesthesiologist all the information she or he needs to protect you.
- Know how to ask questions—about the procedures that will be used, and about anything else that concerns you.
- Know what procedures are available and appropriate for different types of surgery or diagnostic procedures, so you can ask for them if they haven't been offered.

Ask:

- Who will be doing my anesthesia?
- Will that person be present throughout the procedure?
- Who will be assisting, and will the assistant be left in charge at any point? If so, will the anesthesiologist be in the hospital, readily available within a few minutes?

• • •

What Is
Anesthesia Today?

• • •

Over the past century and a half, anesthesia has evolved from a crude practice, in which patients inhaled the vapors of a cloth or sponge soaked in ether or chloroform, into a sophisticated medical specialty. As a result, we are no longer forced to adopt the attitude that pain is an expected, inevitable fact of life. Doctors can now relieve even the most severe, formerly intractable types of pain.

The History of Anesthesia

In the first century C.E., the Roman writer Celsus asserted that the right state of mind for a surgeon was "pitilessness." For centuries, unable to relieve the agonizing pain their patients suffered, surgeons learned simply to ignore it. Before the development of anesthesia, the best they could offer were concoctions that combined opium with whiskey or wine. Other attempts to relieve surgical pain involved hypnosis, herbs, drinking large quantities of alcohol, chewing coca leaves, and local applications of ice or pressure, but all were essentially futile. In 1839 the French surgeon Louis Velpeau remarked, "To obviate pain in operations is a chimera which it is today no longer permissible to seek after."[1]

In less than ten years, he was proved wrong. On October 16, 1846, William T. G. Morton, a New England dentist, gave the first public demonstration of the anesthetizing properties of ether at the Massachusetts General Hospital in Boston. Morton—after experimenting with a pet dog and then successfully anesthetizing dental patients—used an inhaler device to anesthetize Edward G. Abbott, who was having a tumor removed from his neck. Abbott reported that he had remained aware of the procedure but felt no pain. Soon after, Dr. Oliver Wendell Holmes suggested the word "anaesthesia" (from a Greek term meaning "lack of feeling") to describe this state of being temporarily insensitive to pain. News of

Morton's feat spread rapidly, and before long surgeons all over the world began anesthetizing their patients.

The first surgical anesthetics were inhaled drugs, since before the invention of the hypodermic needle and the development of sterile technique, inhalation was the only way effective anesthesia could be provided. Diethyl ether, a volatile liquid, had been known since at least the sixteenth century, when the Swiss physician Paracelsus prepared it by distilling oil of vitriol (sulfuric acid) with fortified wine. He observed that it made chickens fall asleep and also had pain-killing qualities. But its main use until the nineteenth century was as a recreational drug among poor people, who drank it when gin was too expensive.

Nitrous oxide (also known as "laughing gas") was discovered in 1773 by the English scientist Joseph Priestley and studied by chemist Sir Humphry Davy, who noted that it "appears capable of destroying physical pain [and] may probably be used with advantage during surgical operations in which no great effusion of blood takes place." But neither he nor anyone else pursued this possibility, and nitrous oxide too found a use only at parties and public gatherings, where people inhaled it to get high. Still, this application of nitrous oxide and ether did give two Americans the idea that inhaling a vapor could temporarily relieve pain.

In 1842 William E. Clarke and Crawford W. Long both successfully alleviated pain during surgical procedures by administering ether from a soaked towel: the first gave it to a woman having a tooth extracted and the second to a man having a tumor removed. Neither published an account of his procedure, however, so the public glory fell to Morton.

The year after Morton's demonstration, James Y. Simpson, a Scottish obstetrician who had used ether to relieve labor pains, introduced chloroform—a volatile liquid first created in 1831—as a more effective alternative, after inhaling it at a dinner party with a group of friends, all of whom became unconscious. John Snow, a British physician who became the first anesthesiologist, gave Queen Victoria chloroform on a folded handkerchief to ease labor pains during her last two deliveries.

In the decades that followed, other physicians popularized anesthesia and, through experiments and clinical experience, made it safer. Some attempted to administer local anesthesia that would relieve pain at the site of surgery without putting people out. The hollow metal needle was invented in 1853 by the American Alexander Wood, in order to inject morphine into a sensitive part. At the time it was not known that morphine is actually a systemic drug—its action is not confined to a local site but affects the entire body. Thirty years later, however, the hollow needle made possible the use of cocaine (an extract of coca leaves) as the first effective local anesthetic.

Spinal anesthesia, a form of regional anesthesia that affects the spinal cord and the nerves leading out from it, was first performed by neurologist Leonard Corning in 1885 on a dog by anesthetizing its rear legs only. Corning next tried administering cocaine to the lower spinal cord of a man "addicted to masturbation" (then considered a health-threatening vice). In this case, however, the drug did not have the desired effect—though it did produce analgesia that lasted for hours. Not until 1899 was spinal anesthesia given to patients during surgery.

In the twentieth century, pioneering surgeons and anesthesiologists continuously refined their techniques and developed better synthetic anesthetics which solved early problems of incomplete anesthesia, severe headaches, and other complications. Anesthesia became a complex discipline, with the anesthesiologist a specialist distinct from the surgeon who had formerly given anesthesia himself or directed lower-level technicians in providing it.

Types of Anesthesia

Since the early days, the types of anesthesia we use haven't changed much; we continue to give general and regional anesthesia, as well as conscious sedation (administration of drugs that do not make people unconscious but change their perception of pain). But the drugs themselves have changed dramatically, and today we have a wide range available. Our current drugs are much safer for the patient and have fewer side effects than the ether and chloroform of the past, which invariably produced nausea and vomiting and often caused heart abnormalities and degeneration of the liver and kidneys. They were also flammable—a hazard not only for the patient but for the operating room personnel.

Three basic types of drugs are used in anesthesia. An anesthetic provides analgesia, or pain relief. A sedative calms the patient down and induces sleep. A hypnotic, also called an amnestic, causes amnesia—that is, it makes you forget the procedure.

General Anesthesia

We give general anesthesia when loss of consciousness during surgery is desirable—for example, if the patient prefers not to be aware of what's going on. In fact, this is a common reason for using general anesthesia.

Sometimes, too, regional anesthesia is not appropriate for the procedure, as in certain types of brain surgery.

General anesthesia does involve certain risks. First, patients lose protective reflexes, such as the gag and cough reflexes. When these reflexes are lost, the patient might vomit and aspirate (inhale) the vomitus into the lungs, where the stomach acid would irritate the tissue, leading to an inflammation called pneumonitis. Inhaled chunks of food may also block the bronchi or airways, causing them to contract. Bronchospasm, as this contraction is called, prevents the patient from breathing, starving the body tissues of oxygen; it may be fatal.

A second risk is that the ability to breathe decreases significantly under general anesthesia, so the anesthesiologist has to pay close attention to breathing and sometimes even assist the patient's breathing.

General anesthesia consists of three stages: we induce anesthesia with one drug, maintain it with another, and bring you out of it with a third. We often use the sedative thiopental for induction because it's extremely safe, with few side effects. Often referred to as "truth serum," thiopental is given as an intravenous injection and has a very short duration of action of about ten minutes.

Numerous other drugs are available for induction, and we choose them according to their different properties, based on each patient's needs. For example, in patients who are hypertensive (have high blood pressure), thiopental can cause hypotension (low blood pressure). For them we might use another sedative, etomidate. A third sedative, propofol, also causes hypotension, but its duration of action is shorter.

Another way to induce anesthesia is to give certain drugs, such as midazolam, a short-acting amnestic, as a syrup, orally. We often do this with children who fear needles. The drug can also be inserted into the rectum, but this is more uncomfortable than the oral route.

After induction with a sedative, we may need to control the patient's breathing by placing a laryngeal mask airway (LMA) or inserting a breathing tube into the trachea (windpipe). The LMA is a tube with a device at the end that fits like a mask over the opening of the trachea. It's not as reliable as a regular breathing tube, so we use it in simpler procedures. On the other hand, it's less likely to irritate the lining of the trachea and cause necrosis (death of tissue) or bronchospasm.

If insertion of a breathing tube (endotracheal intubation) is necessary, we must administer a drug called a muscle relaxant that blocks nerve receptors on muscles and prevents them from contracting. Paralyzed throat muscles allow the tube to be inserted, while paralysis of the respiratory muscles prevents the patient from coughing on it. Sometimes we also need to use a muscle relaxant when placing an LMA. Muscle relaxants include succinylcholine (short-acting), cisatracurium (intermediate-acting), and pancuronium (long-acting).

Once anesthesia has been induced and muscle paralysis obtained, we generally switch to an inhalation anesthetic, which we provide continuously during the procedure to achieve a level of unconsciousness that prevents you both from feeling pain and from being aware of what's happening during the surgery. Isoflurane, sevoflurane, and desflurane are the most common inhalation drugs used for adults. For children, we use sevoflurane or halothane. (Although halothane may be toxic to the liver in adults, causing a chemically induced form of hepatitis, we haven't seen that effect in children.)

An alternative to inhalation is to maintain general anesthesia by continuous intravenous infusion; this is known as total intravenous anesthesia. In skilled hands, this method is superior to inhalation when it's important to prevent wide variations in blood pressure and heart rate. We induce intravenously, then continue giving anesthesia by this route, switching to different drugs, such as propofol, combined with a continuous infusion of a very potent synthetic narcotic—fentanyl, sufentanyl, alfentanyl, or the very short-acting remifentanil.

Usually, patients who receive inhalant anesthetics have amnesia—that is, they can't remember the surgery—because we can monitor the concentrations of inhalants more precisely. With intravenous anesthetics, however, amnesia is less certain. Patients generally don't feel pain, but they may remember being pushed or pulled or talked about by the operating room staff. To prevent remembering, along with the intravenous anesthetic we give either the amnestic midazolam or a low-dose inhalation anesthetic, which will cause a temporary loss of memory.

Awareness

Very rarely (in no more than 0.2 percent of all cases), a phenomenon called "awareness" occurs under general anesthesia. In one case, a woman who was paralyzed by the muscle relaxant and therefore unable to speak woke up after induction and lived through the nightmare of feeling the entire procedure as her ovaries were removed; her anesthesiologist had forgotten to fill the vaporizer that dispensed the inhalation anesthetic. Sometimes patients who do receive anesthesia have similar experiences. We don't know why this happens, but we think it may be a result of not giving enough anesthesia. Awareness ranges from a sense of one's organs being pushed and pulled about to a conscious experience of actual pain from the surgery. It occurs more often under total intravenous anesthesia, since most of the inhalation anesthetics induce amnesia. The memory of awareness can be distorted by the anesthesia, but certainly for some people it can be devastating.

Currently, it is not standard practice to monitor brain waves during anesthesia to assess the depth of the patient's unconsciousness, for as yet no monitor has been developed that solves the technical problems involved. We do, however, watch for increased heart rate and blood pressure and for sweating; these are signs that the patient feels pain, which means that anesthesia is inadequate.

Painful awareness is more likely to occur in patients who undergo emergency surgery for trauma after losing massive amounts of blood. Because in such cases it is critical to maintain the blood pressure, we must use anesthetics sparingly, if at all, until the bleeding is controlled.

Anesthesia Is Not Sleep

What's the difference between anesthesia and sleep? The brain-wave patterns during general anesthesia and sleep are quite similar. Yet anesthesia and sleep are fundamentally different; anesthesia, unlike sleep, prevents perception of pain and eliminates memory. Unlike sleep, you can't be awakened from anesthesia unless the drug is discontinued. We could say, then, that for a neuron (nerve cell), the difference between sleep and anesthesia is like the difference between rest and paralysis for a muscle.

Whether these differences result primarily from anesthetic drugs intensifying a mechanism that is similar in anesthesia and in sleep, or from qualitative dissimilarities between the two states, we don't know. We believe that general anesthesia affects many areas of the brain, whereas sleep affects only certain areas, such as the reticular activating system, the wakefulness center in the brain stem. Under anesthesia, most of the circuits in the brain are inhibited, so sensory input is blocked. In sleep, by contrast, that input is not completely blocked, which is why a loud noise can awaken you.

There are three basic theories about the mechanisms responsible for these differences. One suggests that anesthetics alter the cell membranes of the neurons to prevent the action of the neurotransmitters (chemicals that carry nerve impulses to and from neurons). A second posits that the drugs interfere with the cell receptors for the neurotransmitters in such a way that the transmission of all impulses, including painful ones, is blocked. A third theory proposes that the drugs change the balance between stimulatory and sleep-producing neurotransmitters so that the latter predominate, producing unconsciousness. These mechanisms are not mutually exclusive; each may play a role.

Regional Anesthesia

Regional anesthesia does not make you unconscious; only the part of the body being operated on is affected, so you remain awake but don't feel pain. A local anesthetic is injected around a major nerve or into the site where a major nerve that supplies an extremity (a leg or an arm) originates at the spinal cord. The major nerves branch off the spinal cord like the branches of a tree, and we give the injection at different levels according to which nerves we want to anesthetize. The anesthetic affects the entire nerve beyond the site of the injection, and all its branches, which means we can anesthetize very specific areas of the body, depending on where we place the shot. We usually also give a sedative and amnestic to decrease patients' level of consciousness. This makes them more comfortable during the procedure.

We use regional anesthesia for patients who wish to remain awake and also when there's a specific medical indication for it. For example, partial removal of the prostate gland is performed by going in through the urethra. During this procedure, called transurethral resection, fluid is continuously infused to wash out the pieces of the prostate, and the body absorbs this fluid. If the patient remains awake, we can assess any changes in his mental status that would indicate a fluid overload.

Regional anesthesia can be difficult to perform, so ask your anesthesiologist how much experience he or she has with the particular type of regional you'll be getting. The best answer would be that the anesthesiologist has performed this procedure numerous times.

The basic types of regional are spinal and epidural anesthesia and nerve blocks.

Spinal Anesthesia

Spinal anesthesia is generally used for people having surgery below the waist. It is easier and quicker to administer than epidural anesthesia and has a higher success rate. We inject a local anesthetic into the fluid surrounding the spinal cord, generally at the second, third, or fourth lumbar vertebra, which means in the upper part of the low back. The needle punctures the dura mater, the outermost of the three membranes that cover the spinal cord and the brain; the dura holds the spinal fluid around the cord.

Spinal anesthesia blocks not only pain, but also the sympathetic nerves that maintain the tone of the blood vessels.(The sympathetic nervous system is part of the autonomic nervous system, which governs involuntary functions; it conducts impulses to organs, glands, and blood vessels.) When these vessels become lax under the drug's influence, the blood returns less quickly to the heart, and the patient may develop hypotension. We prevent this complication by giving a large volume of intravenous fluid before administering the spinal anesthetic. If necessary, we might also give a vasopressor (drug that causes the blood vessels to contract), such as phenylephrine.

Because the dura is punctured in a spinal, on very rare occasions bacteria may be introduced into the cerebrospinal fluid, resulting in an infection called meningitis ("meninges" is the collective term for the membranes covering the spinal cord). We can treat this easily with antibiotics if it's detected early; the symptoms include fever and a stiff neck.

Another complication of spinal anesthesia is the "spinal headache." It's more likely to happen when we need to use a large needle (e.g., for people who are obese or have osteoarthritis of the spine) to administer the anesthetic. The spinal fluid leaks through the hole in the dura; the duration of the headache depends on how much fluid leaks and how long the leak persists. Since the spinal fluid provides a cushion that separates the dura from the brain itself, when this fluid drains off through the hole, the cushion is lost, the dura touches the brain tissue, and pain fibers in the dura create the headache. Keeping the patient lying flat for twelve hours after the procedure may prevent this.

Headaches that do occur are treated with analgesics or by closing the leak with an epidural blood patch. We do this by sterilely withdrawing blood from the patient, then injecting it into the epidural space (the area outside the dura). The blood clots and plugs the hole.

Epidural Anesthesia

With epidural anesthesia the drug is injected into a space between the vertebrae, just outside the dura mater. Like spinal anesthesia, epidural anesthesia is most often given below the waist. Placing an epidural requires greater skill than giving a spinal, and the onset of anesthesia takes longer, up to twenty minutes.

Epidurals are commonly used for analgesia during labor and for cesarean deliveries, as well as for orthopedic procedures such as knee and hip replacements. We may also use it for a lobectomy (partial removal, or resection, of a lung); in this case the injection is placed higher up the spine, between the shoulder blades.

We give an epidural when patients want to be awake, most often for labor and delivery—it enables women to push the baby out better—and to relieve postsurgical pain. A continuous epidural can be placed by threading a plastic catheter (flexible tubular instrument) through the epidural needle and leaving it in place. We can continuously infuse anesthesia through it for two to three days, without fear of complications such as meningitis, because the dura is not punctured.

Epidural anesthesia is also effective for long procedures, since, with the catheter in place, we can either increase the level of anesthesia by raising the dose or give more anesthetic when the first dose starts to wear off.

Another major reason to choose epidural anesthesia is that normally patients who have it don't experience a spinal headache. However, since the epidural needle is much larger than the one used for spinal anesthesia, the dura may be inadvertently punctured and the patient may develop a headache. If the hole in the dura is large, it may need to be closed with an epidural blood patch.

Nerve Blocks

Still another form of regional anesthesia is the nerve block. We inject local anesthetics around the nerve roots, which emerge from the spinal cord and form the major nerves that carry sensory information back to the cord and transmit motor impulses out to enable the rest of the body to move. There are as many types of nerve blocks as there are nerves in the body.

In surgery to correct carpal tunnel syndrome in the wrist, to take one example, we block the axillary nerves (which innervate the arm) by injecting into the armpit area.

Another type of block, the cervical plexus block (the cervical plexus is a network of interconnected nerves at the middle of the neck), may be used for carotid endarterectomy, the removal of fatty plaque from inside the carotid artery, which supplies blood to the brain. For this procedure many anesthesiologists prefer to use regional anesthesia, since if the patient remains awake we can monitor his or her mental status to see that enough blood is getting to the brain.

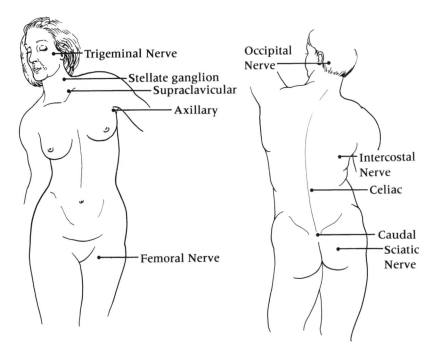

Fig. 1. Locations of major regional blocks.

A caudal block affects the nerve center at the base of the spine. We may use this block for a baby undergoing circumcision, after inducing general anesthesia. The local anesthetic lasts until the procedure is over, relieving pain postoperatively (see chapter 7 for comments on the importance of relieving pain in small children).

Drugs Used for Regional Anesthesia

We choose drugs for regional anesthesia according to the length of the surgical procedure; some local anesthetics may last as long as eight hours, others only forty-five minutes. The anesthetic most frequently used for spinal anesthesia is bupivacaine, whose two- to four-hour duration of action provides enough time to perform hernia repairs and most other procedures. For other forms of regional anesthesia we may use procaine (lasting forty-five minutes), bupivacaine, or other drugs whose duration falls in between, such as ropivacaine, mepivacaine, or lidocaine.

Conscious Sedation and Analgesia

Another form of anesthesia used in stressful diagnostic procedures and some surgical procedures is conscious sedation and analgesia, in which we administer drugs that do not make patients unconscious but change their perception of pain.

Sometimes we need to administer conscious sedation in order to give the regional block; often they're used together. To remove a cataract, for example, the block is placed behind the eye, a procedure so frightening that we administer intravenously a sedative normally used for induction of anesthesia, only in a smaller dose, so the patient remains conscious but sleepy—often not far from general anesthesia.

For an angiogram, a diagnostic procedure that requires threading a catheter through an artery from the groin up into the heart, we first give conscious sedation, then inject a regional block to numb the area. This makes it easier on the patient as a large catheter is inserted into the groin. Once the local anesthetic starts to work, we can lighten the sedation.

Some surgical procedures performed under regional anesthesia require that we place the patient in an unnatural, uncomfortable position. Here again we administer conscious sedation to help the patient tolerate the discomfort.

Conscious sedation and analgesia require maintaining a delicate balance: we must give enough drugs to ensure that patients feel no pain, while also keeping them awake and preventing cessation of breathing. For this reason, an anesthesiologist should always be present.

An eight-year-old boy was referred by a neurologist for an MRI, a diagnostic technique that uses magnetic fields, radio waves, and atomic nuclei to produce cross-sectional images. This procedure requires lying still inside the long tube of a scanner, something even adults often find scary. The boy's mother brought him into the room where the scanner was, and a nurse gave him an injection to sedate him. The child was placed in the tube but began to move around, so the scan could not be done. The nurse returned and repeated the injection. Put back inside the scanner, the child stopped breathing. He had received too much of the sedative drug, which had decreased his respiration. Luckily, the anesthesiologist was nearby and began positive-pressure ventilation (putting a mask on the child's face and using pressure to force air into his lungs) until his breathing returned. Knowing now that the boy was sensitive to sedation, he placed a breathing tube in the child's windpipe and provided mechanical ventilation throughout the procedure.

This incident occurred years ago. Recent federal regulations have made conscious sedation training mandatory for medical personnel working in areas where sedation is given. When problems like this arise, the nurse should be able to save the patient. You should make sure that the personnel present during your procedure have received such training or that an anesthesiologist is present or readily available.

Pain Control

Perhaps the greatest advances in modern anesthesia involve our ability to manage acute and chronic pain. The American Hospital Association now requires that all hospitals state in their patient's bill of rights that they offer both acute and chronic pain management to adult and pediatric patients.

Acute Pain Relief

For the anesthesiologist, acute pain management generally means providing pain relief after surgery. The old idea that it is noble to suffer pain in silence is gradually losing currency, especially since we now know that effective postoperative pain relief is essential for a good recovery; being in pain induces the body to produce hormones that actually impair wound healing.

One method still often used is intramuscular injection of narcotics, injecting the drug into a muscle. Once the patient is able to take medications orally, we give pills instead of injections. The most common form of acute pain relief today, however, is patient-controlled analgesia (PCA). A catheter is placed into a vein and connected to a solution containing a narcotic that is infused by a pump. The patient controls the administration of this infusion by pushing a button when she or he feels pain. The pump is preset to prevent an overdose, and the preset amount can be changed according to the patient's needs.

Clinical studies have shown that patients who can control their own pain relief actually use lower doses of narcotics than those who must ask a nurse for an injection every four to six hours. This is because PCA decreases the anxiety felt by the patient who must wait for an injection—for, as everyone who has been a hospital patient knows, when you press that call button, the nurse is often busy and can't come right away.

A third, very effective form of acute pain relief is epidural patient-administered analgesia. Here again patients receive a pump and can inject themselves through an epidural catheter left in place after surgery.

Injected as little as once a day in this manner, narcotics can provide complete pain relief without interfering with muscle function—unlike intramuscular injection of local anesthetics, which can cause muscle paralysis. Epidural analgesia therefore allows the patient to get up and walk soon after the surgery. Early ambulation, as this is called, helps to prevent deep vein thrombosis, that is, development of a blood clot in a vein in the leg due to inaction, and pulmonary embolism, which occurs when the clot travels to the lung and blocks the circulation there—a complication that can be fatal.

Epidural analgesia also induces dilation of blood vessels, which, by increasing the blood supply, promotes faster healing of the surgical wound. Together, these effects add up to a shorter hospital stay. Finally, epidural analgesia usually does not cause as much nausea and vomiting that all narcotics may induce when given intramuscularly or intravenously. For these reasons I recommend that you request this form of analgesia if it's available. Unfortunately, some hospitals don't provide it, so you may have to take intramuscular injections.

Narcotics and local anesthetics are the drugs usually given for postoperative pain relief. The most frequently used narcotics are morphine sulfate (the form of morphine, a derivative of opium, usually preferred in the United States) and Demerol (meperidine hydrochloride, a synthetic narcotic). In my experience, morphine provides better pain relief, with fewer side effects; Demerol causes a fast heartbeat, which some patients find uncomfortable. However, some patients are allergic to morphine, so they need Demerol. And some physicians just like Demerol; they were trained with it, and feel comfortable using it.

If you have had previous experience with narcotics, don't hesitate to tell your anesthesiologist which one you want. I find that some patients are afraid that if they express a preference the doctor will think they're addicts. But this fear is misplaced. It's important to say what you prefer, so that you can be as comfortable as possible. The doctor understands pain control and will not think you're an addict.

For epidural analgesia, we generally use a long-acting form of morphine. We might also give one of the synthetic narcotics from the fentanyl family, but these drugs have a shorter action; they may last only three to four hours, as opposed to the morphine's twenty-four. The fentanyl narcotics are extremely potent and can cause people to stop breathing if administered intramuscularly or intravenously. For this reason they are used only for epidural analgesia and for intravenous administration of general anesthesia (which is safe because during surgery the anesthesiologist breathes for the patient; see chapter 3 for a description of how this is done).

Chronic Pain Relief

Today patients with chronic pain no longer need to suffer, for a variety of techniques and drugs are available to manage chronic pain syndromes. Generally, we use a multidisciplinary approach in which the anesthesiologist is one member of a pain team that also includes other specialists (see chapter 15 for details). The anesthesiology component of this approach includes temporary and permanent nerve blocks and implantable devices that infuse drugs around nerves or electrically stimulate them.

Nerve Blocks. Nerve blocks can control the pain of terminal diseases such as pancreatic cancer. We use a fluoroscope, a device with a screen on which are projected the shadows of x-rays passing through the body, to visualize the location of the nerves that supply the pancreas. We then inject a local anesthetic into these nerves.

We start by administering a trial block to see if it works. Because the permanent block is a serious procedure that can cause numbness, we need to do at least three trials to be sure that the drug is really effective, not just acting as a placebo. I once treated a woman with a complex regional pain syndrome in her left arm, caused by a fall that stretched the nerves in the arm. We did a block for her and tried to assess whether it was effective, which we do by observing whether the eyelid droops. Her pain was intense, but she insisted the block had relieved it. Yet her eye was normal, which meant the drug had had no physiological action on the involved nerve. Such is the power of the placebo effect.

If the trial block does work, we do a permanent block by injecting phenol, a neurotoxin (which destroys nerve tissue). This block provides pain relief lasting six months to a year.

To relieve various forms of chronic low back pain not caused by nerve damage, we use a different type of block, consisting of injections of a local anesthetic combined with steroids. Generally, after three or four of these injections, given once a week, the pain disappears for an indefinite period. (See chapter 16 for a more detailed discussion of low back pain.) The theory is that when you have chronic pain of this type, a cycle develops in which transmission of pain impulses is no longer inhibited by the specialized nerve cells in the spinal cord that normally block pain transmission. The anesthetic drugs interrupt this pain cycle, allowing the normal inhibition to resume. Another major aspect of chronic pain seems to be an inflammatory response, in which tissue swelling irritates the nerves by exerting pressure on them. At the same time, release of inflammatory chemicals irritates the nerves directly. The steroids act to decrease this response.

Implantable Devices. We can also relieve chronic pain by implanting a tiny pump that continuously infuses small doses of narcotics into the nerves that transmit pain impulses to the brain. This device is effective in cases of ovarian or cervical cancer with metastases into the pelvic area. We insert a catheter into the epidural space and implant the pump under the skin, usually in the abdomen below the belly button. The pump works automatically and can be refilled by injecting more of the drug into it with a needle.

A different implantable device delivers still another form of pain control: electrical stimulation. Wires run under the skin from the stimulator to the area from which the pain impulses are transmitted. The device is set to release a small current that continuously stimulates the nerve fibers in that area. The effect is to inhibit the transmission of pain impulses to the brain. Like a pacemaker for the heart, the stimulator must be removed when the battery needs to be changed. We use it particularly for a condition known as sympathetic dystrophy, in which chronic pain results from degeneration of sympathetic nerves after an injury to an arm or a leg.

Narcotic Patches. For chronic pain in adults, we also use narcotic patches. The patch, which resembles a Band-Aid, is impregnated with the drug. It can be applied anywhere on the skin, and the drug will be absorbed. For example, if you have chronic back pain, a patch will allow systemic absorption of the anesthetic for twenty-four hours. You simply apply a new patch every day. It provides a way to administer a low-dose narcotic without needle punctures or performing a surgical procedure.

Ambulatory Surgery

Ambulatory surgery—so named because you walk in and out of a hospital, a free-standing ambulatory surgery center, or a doctor's office on the same day—is now the most common form of surgery in this country; at least 65 percent of surgical patients have this type of procedure. The popularity of ambulatory surgery arises from the need to decrease costs, along with the realization that patients do better if they can recover at home, in familiar surroundings and with their normal support system (those with no family or friends available to care for them must stay in the hospital until they've completely recovered from all anesthetic effects, which may mean overnight). We've found that the rate of complications after ambulatory procedures is certainly not greater, and may even be smaller, than for procedures involving overnight hospital stays.

What makes ambulatory procedures possible is the shorter duration of new anesthetics and muscle relaxants. The newer anesthetics also have fewer side effects, such as nausea and vomiting, and we also now have drugs that decrease the likelihood of nausea and vomiting in the first place. In addition, technical developments such as laser, fiberoptic, and microscopic surgery have substantially diminished the invasiveness of surgical procedures. The brief stay in the surgical facility, however, requires a great deal of preparation ahead of time.

Preoperative Evaluation

On arrival, you're seen first by your surgeon, who evaluates you and schedules you for surgery. Then your anesthesiologist, or a nurse, sees you, or at least speaks with you on the phone. Depending on your medical condition, the surgeon or anesthesiologist may order lab tests. In the past, we routinely ordered an array of tests, but most ambulatory surgical patients today don't need them. Large studies that have assessed the cost-benefit ratio of routine testing show that it provides no significant benefits. And patients today don't have the time to leave work for separate trips to the doctor, the lab for a blood test, the radiologist for an x-ray, and the cardiologist for an electrocardiogram (EKG, a graphic recording of the electrical activity of the heart).

We generally require no tests unless there's some specific indication for them. For this reason, if you have fatigue, chest pain, a chronic cough, shortness of breath, dizziness, heart palpitations, difficulty walking, weakness, or nausea and vomiting—all signs that preoperative testing might be necessary—you must be sure to tell the anesthesiologist this.

Some time before the day of surgery you'll have seen a member of the nursing staff in the unit where the surgery will be done. Normally, the nurse will instruct you not to eat or drink for six to eight hours before the time the surgery is scheduled, and tell you when to arrive at the unit. The nurse will also give you instructions about discharge after surgery, including the requirement that someone accompany you home afterward.

You should be instructed that if you have a preexisting medical condition, you must continue taking your usual medications on the day of your surgery (with certain exceptions, which I explain below, for the conditions where they apply); otherwise, problems may arise during the procedure, such as a sudden rise in blood pressure.

Choice of Anesthetics

Anesthesia for ambulatory procedures is different from that for longer hospital stays, so it's particularly important to be aware of the risk factors involved.

For ambulatory surgery, we choose anesthetics that are short-acting, with minimal side effects. Since multiple drugs are required for these procedures, we must either select drugs that have minimal interactions with each other or be able to manage the way they are used so that adverse interactions do not occur. For example, the intravenous sedative propofol and the narcotic remifentanyl are ideal for ambulatory surgery because both have a very short duration of action. Used in combination, however, they can result in hypotension. Thus the anesthesiologist must carefully balance the amount of each that is used to avoid this potential adverse effect.

Similarly, when we need to use a muscle relaxant, we must choose one with a short action while also advising the surgeon not to give certain antibiotics whose effects are additive with (that is, increase) those of the muscle relaxant. A stronger action of the muscle relaxant would prolong your recovery period, meaning you might not be able to walk out the same day.

Potential Problems to Be Aware Of

If you or your family have had any previous problems with anesthesia, such as a difficult intubation, difficulty awakening afterward, prolonged nausea and vomiting, memory loss, high fever (over 104°F), or muscle pain, you must be sure to describe them to the anesthesiologist before your surgery, since these are risk factors that, if not taken into account, may lead to your having to remain in the hospital instead of going home the same day.

The same thing might happen if the anesthesiologist is not aware of all the drugs you're taking. For example, if you forgot to mention that you're taking a nonsteroidal anti-inflammatory drug, such as aspirin, for arthritis, you might continue bleeding after the operation and have to remain in the hospital for observation.

Make sure that you aren't discharged before the anesthetics have fully worn off. Normally, the stay is about four hours after the procedure and then you are discharged by a physician. If you have any residual weakness or nausea and vomiting, or cannot urinate, be sure to tell the doctor. A feeling that your eyelids are heavy isn't just sleepiness—it indicates muscle relaxation and is a sign that the anesthesia hasn't worn off. If you've had a regional, be sure you can move your legs well and that they support you without tiring easily before you agree to go home. Make sure feeling has returned to the area that was blocked by the anesthesia, since if this part should touch a hot object you'd be burned without knowing it. Be sure you can urinate, since sometimes the anesthetics interfere with this function.

Same-Day-Admit Surgery

Some patients who will have to remain in the hospital for a time after surgery are nevertheless admitted on the same day that the operation is performed. The initial motivation for this practice was the need to decrease costs by shortening the time patients spend in the hospital, but we've subsequently found that some patients admitted on the day of surgery are less anxious, since they sleep better in their own homes. Since reducing anxiety is an important factor in a successful outcome (see chapter 4), this fact provides support for same-day admittance. Even patients having major surgery—kidney transplants or open-heart and neurosurgery procedures—are now candidates for it. As chapter 4 explains, however, I believe that for patients having such complicated operations anxiety can be better controlled in the hospital.

Since you will arrive at the hospital the day of your surgery, the same guidelines as for ambulatory procedures apply regarding preoperative consultations with the surgeon, anesthesiologist, and nursing staff. However, a same-day-admit patient should be seen in person by the anesthesiologist, since the need for a complete preoperative evaluation is much greater for these complex procedures. In addition, this patient commonly has already had laboratory tests, a chest x-ray, and an EKG.

It's even more important for a same-day-admit patient to tell the anesthesiologist beforehand of any symptoms such as those described above under "Preoperative Evaluation" for ambulatory surgery, since these conditions will need to be looked at in greater detail.

Office-Based Anesthesia and Surgery

Quite recently, surgeons—including plastic surgeons, otolaryngologists, and even some general surgeons—have begun performing surgery in their offices. This is a new development that state health departments have not yet caught up with. An ambulatory surgery center with multiple operating rooms must meet specific safety guidelines mandating the presence of emergency resuscitation equipment and personnel trained in advanced life support. But in most states, a physician may have one operating room adjoining an office without any standards of care, approval, or oversight at all.

Originally, very minor procedures were performed in such facilities, such as removing warts or skin cancers. But soon, doctors began performing more complex operations in their offices, so that currently hemorrhoid removals, face lifts, and even hernia repairs are done in offices. While most such procedures are uneventful, some tragedies have occurred.

In one case, a fifty-two-year-old woman came to a plastic surgeon's office for a complete face lift. The surgeon administered sedation and performed the operation. The only other person present was a nurse who had not been trained to properly monitor the patient and was not aware that sedatives can stop a person's breathing. Early on in the procedure, the surgeon noticed the patient's blood was dark, which meant she wasn't getting enough oxygen. In fact, she had stopped breathing. He began to resuscitate her but couldn't, for he lacked the necessary equipment. Unfortunately, incidents like this happen more often than you might imagine, for every patient responds differently to anesthesia; ideally, the doctor should be prepared for anything.

As a result of events like this woman's death, every state is working with its state anesthesiology and surgical societies to develop standards for office-based surgeries. In the meantime, if you go for a surgical procedure in a doctor's office:

- Ask that an anesthesiologist be present.

If this is not possible, ask:

- Is there someone trained to manage me during conscious sedation? That is, there should be someone other than the physician—two people are necessary—who is certified in advanced life support by the American Heart Association.
- Do you have a defibrillator (device to counteract irregular heartbeats) and a crash cart with emergency drugs and respiratory support equipment, in case a complication arises?

Ideally, an anesthesiologist should be present. It's safer to have one, and there are plenty around.

Whether ambulatory or same-day-admit, shorter hospital stays—generally known as "fast-tracking"—as well as office-based procedures will become increasingly common, driven not only by the need for cost reduction but by patients' desire to be at home. The fact is, people don't really need to be in the unfamiliar, and essentially unhealthy, environment of a hospital, where mistakes are made by overworked staff and patients are exposed to potentially severe infections. I have found that as long as you make sure you've adequately recovered from surgery and don't let them push you out too soon, you can get well much better at home. What is important is that you, the patient/consumer, be an active, aware participant in your own care before, during, and after surgery.

Summary: Questions and Points to Remember

- Is there someone—preferably an anesthesiologist—trained to manage me during conscious sedation?

For ambulatory procedures:

- Do you have a defibrillator (device to counteract irregular heartbeats) and a crash cart with emergency drugs and respiratory support equipment, in case a complication arises?
- Ask that an anesthesiologist be present.

NOTE

1. Quotations and information on the history of anesthesiology are from Rod K. Calverley, "Anesthesiology as a Specialty: Past, Present, and Future," in Paul B. Barash, Bruce F. Cullen, and Robert K. Stoelting, *Clinical Anesthesia*, 3d ed. (Philadelphia and New York: Lippincott-Raven, 1997), 3–11.

CHAPTER 3

• • •

What Does the
Anesthesiologist Do?

• • •

When I first saw Bob in our hospital, my initial impression was of how large he was: six feet five and three hundred pounds. Though robust looking, Bob, who was forty-six, was in considerable distress, with severe pain in his abdomen and back. He'd been referred by our vascular surgeon because he had an aneurysm, a pouch that had formed in the dilated wall of his aorta, the major artery that carries blood from the heart. If the weakened arterial wall ruptured, massive bleeding and death would follow.

Bob had already been admitted, so his blood pressure, pulse, respiration rate, height, and weight had been taken and recorded. Upon examining him, I found his skin cold, heartbeat and breathing rapid, and blood pressure high. His abdomen was distended, which indicated a mass within it—the aneurysm. Clearly, speed was critical: Bob needed to be operated on before the aneurysm ruptured.

After completing the exam, I reviewed the lab tests the surgeon had ordered. We needed to see whether his blood count was low, which would indicate that blood was leaking from the aneurysm into his abdomen. His potassium level was important, since his high blood pressure had been treated with a drug that has a side effect of lowering potassium. Since low potassium can cause heart abnormalities and even cardiac arrest, he might need a potassium supplement. Since Bob also had arteriosclerosis, or hardening of the arteries, an electrocardiogram (EKG) had been ordered to determine whether he had cardiac ischemia (decreased blood supply to the heart) or abnormal heartbeats, which would have to be treated before surgery.

He also had a chest x-ray, to rule out any other abnormalities in the chest area, and a urinalysis. Blood in his urine would indicate that the aneurysm was close to the renal arteries, which supply the kidneys. If this was the case, I would need to pay even more attention to his urine output throughout the operation. Finally, his arterial blood gas—the concentration of oxygen and carbon dioxide in aerated blood coming from the heart—was measured to determine whether his respiration was impaired. If so, I'd know to devote special care to breathing for him during the procedure.

When the lab results came back an hour later, I saw that Bob's potassium level was indeed low. I gave him a potassium supplement, administered through an intravenous catheter that had already been placed. He was scheduled for urgent surgery that same afternoon.

Bob was given a sedative to keep him from becoming anxious—which, by raising his blood pressure, could cause the aneurysm to rupture—as well as drugs to control his blood pressure. Another large intravenous catheter was placed in a vein in the back of his nondominant hand to provide easy access for inducing anesthesia and for infusing fluids and blood if needed.

Before his operation, Bob was given his usual medications orally—omitting them could have worsened his condition—and brought to the operating room. Here he was put in a quiet, comfortable holding area, and the first group of monitors to be used during his surgery were placed.

The number of these monitors will give you an idea of how complex a discipline anesthesia can be for serious operations like Bob's. He had a special EKG with five electrodes that were placed on his chest so that the entire heart could be monitored for ischemia. We inserted an arterial catheter in his wrist just above the thumb. This catheter was connected to a transducer that translated the strength of the heartbeat into an electrical signal, to provide beat-to-beat monitoring of his blood pressure as blood pumped through the artery. Another catheter, called a Swan-Ganz or pulmonary artery catheter, was inserted into a vein in his neck and run down through the right side of his heart into its left side, the side that pumps oxygenated blood from the lungs out into the body. The pulmonary artery catheter monitors fluid volume and left heart function, permitting rapid treatment of sudden loss of fluid and heart ischemia, which otherwise would lead to death of heart tissue.

During the procedure, if Bob's blood pressure became too low or too high, I would administer drugs that either contracted or relaxed the blood vessels to correct the pressure; if I saw changes in his heart rate, I would inject drugs to stabilize it. All this would be done through the catheter in the back of his hand or through the pulmonary artery catheter.

While these monitors were being placed, I gave Bob intravenous midazolam as a sedative, to further decrease anxiety. Now the surgeon came to see him, and together we transported Bob into the operating room

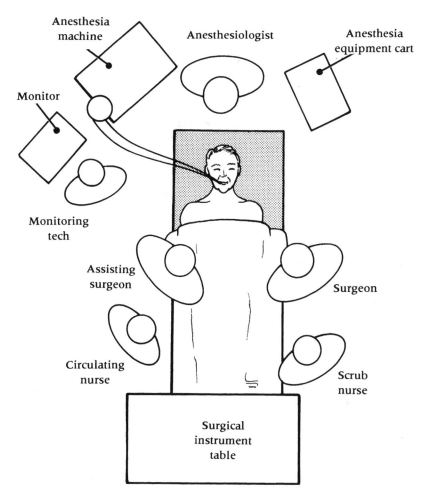

Fig. 2. Bird's-eye view of operating room.

itself. Here he was made comfortable with more blankets and connected to the central monitoring stations so that the surgeon and I could observe his vital signs throughout the procedure: blood pressure, heartbeat, oxygen, carbon dioxide, and the level of anesthetic gases coming from his lungs.

A complex procedure like this requires about seven staff members. In this case, the surgeon was assisted by a physician assistant and I by an anesthesia assistant. (Residents—specialist doctors in training—and nurse anesthetists may also assist during surgery.) The nursing department

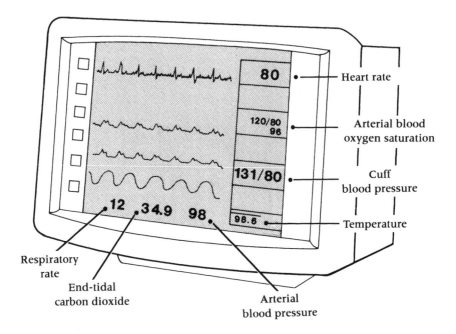

Fig. 3. Anesthesia machine monitor. It can track all necessary vital functions.

provided a scrub nurse and a circulating nurse, who coordinated operating room nursing care and obtained needed supplies. And finally, there were technicians to run the monitors and troubleshoot for technical difficulties.

I planned an intravenous induction, using thiopental, chosen because of its rapid onset and tendency to reduce blood pressure, which I injected into the intravenous catheter in Bob's hand. Now I began to breathe for him; I put a mask over his mouth and forced air into his lungs by squeezing a reservoir bag full of oxygen flowing from the anesthesia machine, which stood to my right.

In addition to a mechanical ventilator (ventilation is the process of breathing in and out), this machine contains connections for delivering compressed gases, valves to control pressure, flowmeters, vaporizers, and monitoring devices. A set of tubes called the breathing circuit runs from the machine to the patient. Through these tubes the patient receives oxygen and inhalant anesthetics. We also use the breathing circuit to measure the levels of carbon dioxide and anesthetic gases as they move in and out of the patient. Other tubes deliver intravenous fluids, including blood, from an IV pole.

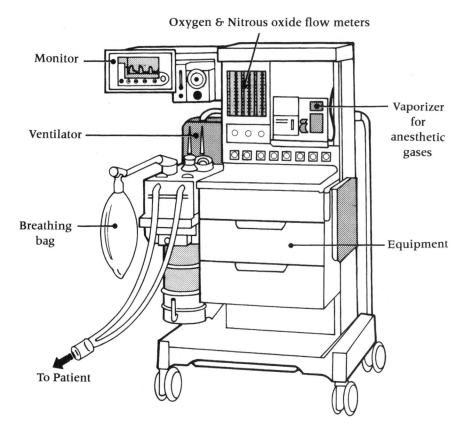

Fig. 4. Anesthesia machine.

A number of drugs—to constrict or dilate the blood vessels, to slow the heart, and so on—are kept on the anesthesia machine. In addition, a cart to my left was loaded with about forty other drugs, as well as equipment needed in most situations that might arise. The most commonly needed drugs lay ready to hand in syringes.

I found it easy to ventilate Bob, which indicated that it was time to give him rocuronium, a long-acting muscle relaxant, which I injected intravenously. We placed a neuromuscular monitor on his left arm to ascertain when he became paralyzed; this generally takes three to five minutes. Meanwhile, I injected the narcotic drug fentanyl intravenously to increase the depth of analgesia, as a preparation for the surgical incision.

Once muscle relaxation was complete, I began to place an endotracheal tube down through Bob's trachea, or windpipe, so that from now on his breathing would be controlled mechanically by the respirator. But here I ran into a difficulty: I couldn't see the opening into the trachea. After several attempts, I asked for a fiberoptic laryngoscope. This is a long, thin tube with glass or plastic fibers running through it and a light at the bottom. It projected an image of the interior of Bob's trachea onto a video screen so I could observe what happened as I pushed the end of the tube downward. What I found was an anatomical anomaly: the opening into his trachea was further forward than normal. With the aid of the video image, however, I was able to place the tube properly, into the upper part of the trachea. The tube had an inflated cuff on it; if Bob vomited, the cuff would prevent aspiration of vomitus into his lungs. I was careful not to overinflate the cuff, since that could injure the trachea and cause breathing problems postoperatively.

More monitors followed. The surgeon placed another catheter, called a Foley catheter, up through Bob's urethra (the canal through which urine flows out of the body) into his bladder to continuously monitor his urine output. If the aneurysm or the surgery interfered with the renal arteries, the volume of urine he produced would drop. I placed an esophageal stethoscope through Bob's mouth down into his esophagus, to a point just behind his heart. I would listen continuously through the stethoscope to

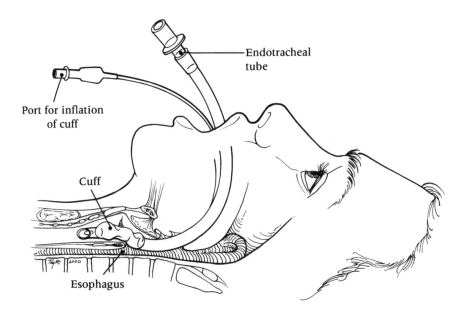

Fig. 5. Endotracheal intubation.

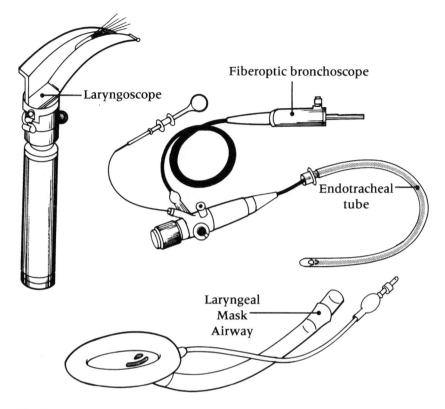

Fig. 6. Equipment used to manage airways.

Bob's heart and breath sounds, in case there was a problem with his ventilation. Connected to the stethoscope was a temperature monitor. (In other procedures, temperature might be measured with a tympanic membrane probe, placed into the ear canal, or, rarely, a rectal probe.)

Next we put a pulse oximeter on Bob's index finger. This device consists of a clamp or fiberoptic patch with a light that passes through the finger. The amount of light transmitted is recorded on the other side and converted to a number showing the amount of oxygen in the blood. We placed an end-tidal carbon dioxide monitor at the end of the breathing circuit, where it connected to the endotracheal tube, to measure the amount of carbon dioxide flowing out of Bob's lungs at the end of each breath. Together, all these respiratory monitors analyze the contents of the airflow and tell us when something is off balance: too much carbon dioxide, too little oxygen, too much anesthetic. An alarm is set on each monitor to go off if any of the preset parameters change significantly.

We also set up a machine called a cell saver for salvaging Bob's blood. The surgeon suctions the blood directly into the machine, which washes it, ridding it of debris so it can be reinfused into the patient whenever necessary during the operation. This is preferable to a transfusion of someone else's blood, which might contain viruses or elicit an allergic reaction.

Finally, we placed an evoked potential monitor, with stimulating electrodes on Bob's foot as well as recording electrodes on his head and at various levels on his spinal cord and lower brain. The monitor measures the speed with which a nerve impulse produced in response to an electrical stimulus to the foot travels up the spinal cord to the brain. Since aneurysm repair sometimes interrupts the blood flow to the cord (which could cause permanent paralysis), it's important to monitor for abnormalities in spinal cord function—indicated by a delay in the length of time required for the nerve impulse to travel to the brain. If a problem occurred, I would administer a drug to raise Bob's blood pressure or tell the surgeon to remove a clamp on an artery, to increase the blood flow to the cord.

At this point I began giving Bob fentanyl as a continuous infusion through the catheter in his hand, while also adding isoflurane as an inhalation anesthetic, delivered from the anesthesia machine through the breathing tube. I chose isoflurane because I could adjust the dose to control Bob's blood pressure better than with fentanyl alone. Isoflurane would also ensure amnesia, since the fentanyl would not block recall of the surgery.

I decided to give Bob fentanyl as an epidural anesthetic as well. To place the epidural catheter in the upper part of his lower back, we turned Bob onto his side, pulled his knees to his chest, and moved his head down. Whereas the IV fentanyl was systemic—that is, it affected Bob's whole body, instead of just the region involved in the surgery—the epidural fentanyl would block transmission of pain impulses locally at the spinal nerve roots, allowing me to give Bob less IV fentanyl and inhaled isoflurane. The epidural catheter would remain in place for up to three days after surgery to provide pain relief. I could have used a local anesthetic instead of epidural fentanyl, but I preferred the narcotic to avoid the effect that the local has of limiting Bob's ability to move after surgery.

With all the monitors in place, the surgeon made a small incision to allow me to assess the degree of anesthesia. There was no increase in Bob's heart rate or blood pressure, which meant anesthesia was adequate, so the surgeon proceeded. He began to open Bob's abdomen, working cautiously since the opening would release abdominal pressure, that might result in rupture of the aneurysm. Happily, this did not occur, and he placed a clamp across the aorta to block the blood flow into the aneurysm while he repaired it. Before he placed the clamp, however, I started an infusion of nitroglycerin—a vasodilator, or drug that causes blood vessels to dilate—to counteract the considerable increase in blood pressure that the clamp would cause. As the repair proceeded, the surgeon was careful to avoid the arteries supplying the spine and the kidneys. Meanwhile, I infused more nitroglycerin to keep Bob's blood pressure down and gave him a diuretic to increase his urine output, which had dropped.

When the repair was completed, I stopped the nitroglycerin and administered a large amount of saline solution. I also had ready vasopressors (the opposite of vasodilators, they cause blood vessels to contract), since removing the clamp on the aorta results in a sharp drop in blood pressure. In both clamping and unclamping the aorta, the pulmonary artery catheter is critically important, for it tells me whether the patient's fluid volume is adequate and whether the heart is overstressed.

When the aorta was unclamped, the EKG monitor showed that Bob's heart was developing ischemia, and the pulmonary artery catheter confirmed this. It also showed that his fluid volume was too low. We therefore infused the salvaged blood. I administered more fluids, a vasopressor, phenylephrine, to raise his blood pressure, and more nitroglycerin, which would both help the heart pump better and help raise the blood pressure. His vital signs returned to normal, and the rest of the surgery proceeded without problems.

After the surgeon closed Bob's abdomen, I injected a long-acting type of morphine through the epidural catheter. This drug would provide analgesia for up to twenty-four hours.

I discontinued the anesthetics, then gave Bob two more drugs: neostigmine, to reverse the effect of the muscle relaxant, and glycopyrolate, to prevent the side effects of neostigmine, particularly slow heartbeat (bradycardia).

Once the anesthetics are stopped and the monitors show that little, if any, anesthetic gases are being exhaled, patients usually awaken. Accordingly, Bob began to make uncoordinated movements; he opened his eyes and gagged on the endotracheal tube. Before I could remove the tube and let him breathe on his own, however, several indicators had to be present. Bob had to be able to respond to verbal commands and to breathe spontaneously at a sufficient rate and with a large enough volume of air passing in and out of his lungs to maintain adequate oxygenation of his blood without assistance.

So I said, "The operation's over, everything's fine. We'll take the tube out as soon as you breathe for me. So take a deep breath." He did; he was awake, with his eyes open, and the monitor showed he was maintaining his oxygenation without my help. I therefore deflated the cuff on the tube and gave him 100 percent oxygen, suctioned the back of his throat, and, still giving him oxygen, removed the tube.

We continued to give him oxygen as we transferred him to the recovery room with his monitors hooked up to a portable readout device. Once he was there, the monitors were connected to a permanent readout monitor. The recovery room was close to the operating room, so that if a problem developed, such as bleeding or a need to reinsert the breathing tube, we could get him back there quickly. Checking all Bob's vital signs once more, I left the nurse a history of the surgery and anesthetics used and turned him over to the anesthesiologist who supervised the recovery room. Bob was closely observed to be sure that his breathing remained adequate, he was not bleeding from the site of surgery, his urine output was steady, and he was able to move his legs. He remained stable, and an hour later, after a discussion with the surgeon, he was discharged from the recovery room and transferred to the intensive care unit, where close supervision of his condition continued.

Within four hours Bob was sitting up in bed—pain free, thanks to the epidural catheter. The staff encouraged him to breathe deeply to prevent atelectasis (collapse of the lungs), which could lead to pneumonia, and to sit up beside his bed. Sitting up was crucial, for it stimulated increased blood flow, promoting wound healing. If problems occurred, I'd be notified, but otherwise I normally see patients the day after surgery to check for any problems they might be having.

When I visited the next morning, Bob was agitated, complaining about the Foley catheter and about not knowing what was going on. I checked his record and spoke to the surgeon and the nurses, who allowed the catheter to be removed.

"Everything's going well," we told him. "You should be able to walk today and possibly go home in two days." He was much relieved; I could see the stress leave his face.

Reassurance, I've learned, is an extremely important element of care. Making rounds in the morning, I notice that when physicians go by, look at the numbers on the charts, but don't talk to patients, the patients become more agitated. But when the first thing the doctor does is communicate, the patient feels greatly relieved.

- You or a friend or family member should insist that the anesthesiologist communicate with you after surgery.

Make sure you keep written notes of these discussions, so that if another anesthesiologist becomes involved in your care, you can repeat to him or her the discussions you had with the first anesthesiologist.

Within two days, Bob was discharged from the intensive care unit (ICU) to a regular hospital unit. On the third day, the rest of his monitors were removed, and he got the last injection of narcotic into the spinal catheter, which was also removed. As he was being prepared for discharge, his surgeon and I instructed him to continue his blood pressure medications and gave him a three days' supply of morphine to take orally after the epidural narcotic wore off, plus a prescription for Tylenol with codeine for the following three days. Eventually, he recovered completely and returned to his normal life.

Bob's case, as I said, was an extremely complex one, which I chose because it illustrates everything the anesthesiologist must be prepared to do. Most patients' problems are far less complicated—though no less important—and they require much less care.

The Anesthesiologist as Critical Care Specialist

Although I visited Bob in the ICU to check that he was okay, another anesthesiologist—an intensive or critical care specialist—was actually in charge of his care there.

The critical care specialist manages all aspects of the care of critically ill patients: intensive postoperative care, trauma care, and care of severe medical conditions, such as respiratory failure. Critical care specialists are prepared to resuscitate patients who develop shock (loss of blood volume and pressure) from various causes, such as blood loss, heart failure, and sepsis (severe, systemic infection). Often various specialists work in the ICU: surgeons, internists, pediatricians, neonatologists, and pulmonologists. Care of ICU patients involves specialized monitoring and procedures, such as placement of transvenous pacemakers (which are inserted through a vein to pace the heart). To be a critical care specialist, a physician needs an additional year or two of training in at least five of the six types of intensive care units: medical, surgical, neurosurgical, pediatric, neonatal, and cardiothoracic (involving the heart and lungs).

In addition to the critical care function of life support, the anesthesiologist is uniquely qualified to provide pain relief in the ICU (see the example in the next section).

Resuscitation after Trauma

I have not devoted an entire chapter to the anesthesiologist's role in the care of injuries, since trauma is generally an emergency situation that does not allow for advance preparation and exercise of choice by the patient. Still, a survey of the anesthesiologist's role in medicine would not be complete without some mention of trauma anesthesiology.

People who sustain severe trauma require immediate resuscitation—that is, procedures to stabilize vital functions such as breathing, heart rate, and blood pressure. The anesthesiologist, along with the emergency medicine specialist, may perform this role in the emergency room, then follow the patient into the operating room for surgery and finally to the intensive care unit, all the while continuing to resuscitate the patient. The anesthesiologist is the airway management expert, who determines whether there is any obstruction in the trachea preventing the injured person from breathing, then clears the airway to ensure that ventilation is adequate, usually by inserting an endotracheal tube.

The anesthesiologist and the emergency medicine doctor are also responsible for replenishing lost fluid volume, for avoiding the need for blood transfusion using a cell saver, and for choosing anesthetics that will be least likely to lower blood pressure further. In the ICU, the anesthesiologist's knowledge of the case is often particularly useful in handling problems that arise postoperatively.

For example, a man who sustained multiple fractures after an auto accident was in the operating room for twelve hours, then was transferred to the ICU, where he complained of severe pain. His wife called the nurse, asking for a painkiller. But the nurse responded that since he had just had anesthesia, pain medication might make him stop breathing. So his wife asked for a critical care doctor. This physician, an anesthesiologist, checked the patient's chart, found he had received inhalation anesthetics with a small amount of narcotics, and ordered IV narcotics, knowing that this treatment would not stop his breathing. Both the patient and his wife fell asleep, relieved.

- If you feel that you, or a family member, aren't getting adequate pain relief, ask for a critical care anesthesiologist or someone with experience in acute postoperative pain management.

After many years as an anesthesiologist, I still experience tremendous satisfaction upon completing a complex treatment like Bob's. Part of this satisfaction comes from feeling, when I go home in the evening, that I've provided life-saving care and pain relief that I'd want available for my own family or friends. Through this book, I hope to help other people access such care.

Summary: Questions and Points to Remember

- You or a friend or family member should ask that the anesthesiologist communicate with you after surgery.
- If you feel that you, or a family member, aren't getting adequate pain relief, ask for a critical care anesthesiologist or someone with experience in acute postoperative pain management.

CHAPTER 4

• • •

Negotiating Managed Care

• • •

Early one evening, my friend Joan developed acute appendicitis and was rushed to a hospital for surgery. She awakened in the recovery room in searing pain, unable to speak or even open her eyes. Had she had a gun, she told me later, she would have shot herself. Around midnight, she was transferred to a bed in the surgical unit, where she spent a restless, sleepless night. At 6:30 the next morning, a nurse appeared and announced that she was preparing Joan for discharge.

Joan objected that she was exhausted and still in pain. The nurse insisted that she had to leave because her managed care company would not pay for another day in the hospital. But Joan resisted. She simply refused to leave, and later that day pulled herself together despite her pain, telephoned the managed care company, and managed to reach some functionary, who asked, "Are you in pain?" When she said, "Yes," he responded that, of course, she could stay.

Joan's pain and her difficulty moving after her surgery were probably the result of the anesthesiologist's having used a combination of short-acting anesthetics and a longer-acting muscle relaxant. The anesthetic would wear off quickly to make an early discharge possible, while the muscle relaxant would stick around, leaving her muscles still weak. Her experience is a classic example of life under managed care. What's important is that when she refused to knuckle under and made a fuss, she got what she needed.

In today's radically changed medical environment, you need to be your own advocate. One aspect of self-advocacy is demanding what you need, as Joan did. (Her experience, by the way, shows how critical it can be to keep your insurance ID always with you, so you have the contact phone number.) Another is asking the right questions beforehand. Asking questions is crucial for two reasons. First, as I explained in the introduction, that is how you get the best care. But an even more important reason to gather as much information as possible about your anesthesia and surgery in advance is that it will reduce your anxiety level.

Being anxious stimulates the body to boost its production of hormones, such as adrenaline, that increase heart rate and blood pressure, and also of hormones, such as cortisol, that decrease your immune system's ability to fight off infection. Extreme anxiety can significantly diminish your chances of a problem-free recovery.

Anyone facing surgery is bound to feel some anxiety, but the best way to minimize it is to know what questions to ask about the particular surgical procedure you'll be having—and then to ask them and get answers. The specific questions will vary considerably, depending on whether you're having minor surgery, such as hernia repair or removal of a mole, or a major procedure, like open-heart surgery. Anesthesia for each surgical subspecialty has unique aspects that must be addressed. The chapters in part 2 will list the questions specific to each medical procedure described. This chapter provides general questions that apply to any procedure involving anesthesia or conscious sedation and analgesia. These questions cover important issues that doctors often don't think about until the patient asks.

The Impact of Managed Care

Ten years ago, I normally saw a patient at least three times before I induced anesthesia for that patient in the operating room. The surgeon would refer to me a man having open-heart surgery, for example. I'd see him first in my office, where I'd go over his history, do a physical examination, review any lab tests he'd already had, and order additional tests I considered necessary. The results of these tests would come back before the patient was admitted to the hospital, so if any results were abnormal—for example, if his blood pressure was too high—I could refer him for treatment during a second office visit or on the phone.

I'd next see this patient in the hospital on the day before surgery, to make last-minute treatment choices or order still more tests if his condition had changed since his last office visit. I could order sleep-inducing and anxiety-relieving drugs, so he could have a restful night before surgery and arrive in the operating room the next morning rested and free of anxiety.

After surgery, the patient would remain in the recovery room until his vital signs were stable. Usually, he stayed there overnight, then was transferred to the ICU, and, after a few days, to a step-down unit for a period of recovery before going home. Today, the first time I see a patient having open-heart surgery is often in the operating room, where he's just arrived from home. Most likely, he's anxious and exhausted from his trip to the hospital very early in the morning. (Bob, in the previous chapter, did spend the night before surgery in the hospital; but this was unusual and happened because his condition was so serious.) It's only then that I get to review the patient's chart, including whatever lab tests the surgeon has ordered, and begin my examination.

As I ask my questions, the patient usually becomes even more anxious, since this is his first opportunity to question me. And, as you can imagine, lying on a stretcher moments before surgery is not the time for anyone to be collected enough to remember everything he wanted to ask—nor to have the opportunity to do something about it if he doesn't like one of my answers. If I conclude from my review of his case that everything is all right, I place the monitors and then administer a sedative through the intravenous line—which finally calms the patient's anxieties.

Sometimes I decide that everything's not okay. The lab tests may be abnormal, or I notice that he's developed excessive fatigue on the way to the hospital, and discover in questioning him that he has a history of asthma and wheezing in the morning. Then the surgery has to be delayed so we can bring the asthma under control. If all is well, on the other hand, the surgery proceeds.

Postoperatively, treatment is now geared to early discharge. This policy obliges me to use anesthetic drugs that are short-acting and allow the vital signs to return quickly to normal. Consequently, some patients—Joan would have been one, if she hadn't fought back—have to leave the hospital while still in pain and still weak from the muscle relaxants. Their anxiety level shoots up, impairing their immune function and possibly resulting in delayed healing and development of infection in the surgical wound.

Today, even after complex operations, the breathing tube is removed while still in the operating room. Often the recovery room is bypassed and the patient goes directly to the ICU, where most of the monitors are removed that day or the next. Two days later, she's prepared for discharge. The pain-relieving drugs she's been receiving in the hospital are replaced by less potent drugs to take at home, which may be less effective. Because of the possible complications that could develop, we can't prescribe the more effective painkillers for home use.

This speeded-up process is known as fast-tracking. It is the consequence of managed care and, more particularly, of managed health care companies negotiating what are called bundled carve-out contracts with hospitals and physicians. Under this type of arrangement, a managed care company negotiates with a hospital and its physicians to handle all cases of a certain type of procedure. For example, the company agrees to send all its open-heart-surgery patients to that hospital, and to pay a specified flat fee for all the care these patients require—whether they need reoperation, how many times they see their doctors, and so on. All the health services for open-heart surgeries, from preop to postop procedures, are bundled together, carved out of the contract, and assigned to this hospital. The inclusive rate covers not only all hospital services but also the professional fees to the surgeon, anesthesiologist, radiologist, and so on.

In negotiating these contracts, the insurance companies pit hospitals against physicians—and sometimes physicians against each other—in a bidding process where the lowest bidders win. The hospitals balance the added volume of business against the reduced fees, evening out the balance by decreasing the amount of care they give through fast-tracking, eliminating preoperative visits, same-day surgery, and the like.

The practical meaning of this arrangement is that the less care patients get, the more money the hospital and doctors make. And since doctors receive no payment for any additional visits, they feel pressure not to have unnecessary contact with patients. In addition, an anesthesiologist or surgeon might not be able to see that open-heart-surgery patient for a preoperative consultation because the contract significantly increases the number of patients who must be seen each day, which means there simply isn't enough time.

Another important consequence is that the anesthesiologist's ability to reduce the patient's anxiety has diminished, both before and after surgery (and, of course, the same is true for other physicians). My experience tells me that being able to ask questions and get answers and reassurance from me decreases patients' anxiety level tremendously. In the past, when I saw patients in the recovery room, I could assure them that all had gone well, and that whatever pain or abnormalities they might be experiencing were normal postoperative reactions. This anxiety reduction played a real role in their recovery. But under fast-tracking, that transition period in the recovery room before the patient is sent to the ICU no longer exists. (Joan was not fast-tracked; that's why she did spend time in the recovery room.)

It's true that for many patients, there's a positive side to fast-tracking. Often anxiety can be most easily relieved by a reassuring family member, so for some patients, spending the night before surgery at home can be preferable to being in the hospital. In my experience, however, patients who are in the hospital, sedated, and given antianxiety drugs are better prepared on the morning of surgery for complex surgical procedures.

Again, while patients may prefer going home soon after surgery instead of staying in the often depressing environment of the hospital, early discharge of patients who are still recovering from serious surgery may make family members anxious, because they now have so much responsibility for the patient's care. Patients often pick up on these feelings, and their own anxiety doubles. The result is release of those hormones that prevent wound healing, depress the immune system, and possibly lead to infections.

So each patient is different; some may benefit more from the old way, and some from the new. There's no doubt, however, that the decreased contact we now have with patients is a loss.

As this discussion indicates, doctors and patients have similar problems with managed care companies. Still, the patient's overriding need is to get the best care—which means that, although in many ways patients and doctors are aligned as allies against the companies, there are times when a patient has to advocate for him- or herself against a doctor. In managed care, physicians are harmed in terms of money and time; they are paid less to see many more patients. For patients, however, life itself can be at stake. Sometimes, therefore, the circumstances of health care today make doctors and patients adversaries.

Given this situation, how can you maximize the care you get?

Insist on a Preoperative Consultation

First of all, if you're having elective surgery, discuss it ahead of time with an insurance company representative so that you know exactly what your plan covers. After that, the most important action you can take is to make sure you have some kind of preoperative consultation with your anesthesiologist, even if it's just over the phone. Once you've arranged it, you need to make the most of it.

Ask your surgeon to schedule you to see your anesthesiologist in advance of surgery. If you have difficulty getting an appointment, keep insisting. If you'll be having a sufficiently complicated procedure, the surgeon will likely want to maximize the chances of success and will ask the anesthesiologist to see you. And if you make enough of a fuss, the anesthesiologist will do so, because anesthesiologists work with surgeons and recognize the need for teamwork. Besides, the anesthesiologist may want more referrals from that surgeon. Should the anesthesiologist not have time to see you, he or she may refer you to another doctor, which is fine.

If you have a serious medical problem, such as asthma, ask your surgeon to refer you not only to an anesthesiologist but also to an internist. Asthma requires close monitoring and treatment before surgery and anesthesia, since anxiety increases the risk of an asthmatic attack. Your medications should be adjusted to treat infections and stop wheezing, if possible. Asthmatics having major elective surgery, such as an abdominal hysterectomy, may require two weeks of treatment before the operation. Frequently, you have to get your surgeon or anesthesiologist to intervene and call the managed care company to obtain an appointment with a participating provider.

Diabetics are another group who need special presurgical care from an internist, since surgery and anesthesia increase the need for insulin. Often, people who haven't recently seen a primary care doctor need to see one before surgery, since the need for surgery means their condition has changed.

If, on the other hand, your condition isn't serious and the procedure is relatively simple, you may be willing—depending on your anxiety level—to wait and see the anesthesiologist on the day of surgery. However, if you really want to speak to the anesthesiologist, you should insist; perhaps you would feel satisfied with a phone conversation instead of a face-to-face meeting. In some hospitals, you may be given a questionnaire to fill out and then be seen by a nurse practitioner or physician assistant (physician assistants are trained to assist in surgery and perform preoperative and postoperative care). This is perfectly fine, if the procedure you'll be having is not complicated or if you have no abnormalities or preexisting medical conditions.

- Ask to see an anesthesiologist prior to surgery if your surgery will be complicated—or simply because you want to.

In my hospital, we still see patients at least two weeks before surgery. Sometimes our preadmission testing unit sees thirty to sixty patients a day for preoperative consultations. I'm quite aware that the more time I spend with one patient, the less I have with the others. Another factor I must add to the balance is that the hospital does patient satisfaction surveys, and if patients have to wait too long, the anesthesia department looks bad. Managed care companies frequently request these surveys before deciding to award contracts.

Thus the pressures on anesthesiologists are complicated, requiring sound judgment to identify patients in need of extra preoperative attention. In my own case, given these constraints, the patients who wind up getting more of my time are either those who are sicker or those who demand it because of their anxiety and their involvement in their own care.

Prepare for the Meeting

Once you've scheduled an appointment, make sure the surgeon's office sends the anesthesiologist a copy of your medical records. Your concise and accurate medical history is critically important and may save your life. You own your medical records. Request them. If you have a complicated medical history that may not all be included in the surgeon's notes, write it down yourself before seeing the anesthesiologist and bring it with you. Not only will it ensure that the anesthesiologist is aware of all your medical problems, but if another anesthesiologist becomes involved in your case, that doctor will have these notes to refer to.

Before the meeting, make a list of the questions you want answered. Write them down. Often when people are on the spot with the doctor, they forget some of the important ones (this goes for phone consultations as well as meetings). Keep in mind that the purpose of asking questions is to decrease your anxiety so as to give yourself the best chance for recovery. Therefore:

- Be sure to prepare questions about *anything* that is making you anxious.

What to Tell the Anesthesiologist

At this meeting, the anesthesiologist will have your records, including lab tests. You should be prepared to supply information about any previous surgeries and any complications you may have had with those surgeries. Also tell the anesthesiologist if someone in your family has died from anesthesia or had a major problem during surgery, such as a high fever. These reactions could represent a genetic abnormality called malignant hyperthermia, which can result in death if unanticipated and untreated. Knowing this history, the anesthesiologist can be prepared and prevent such problems.

Tell the anesthesiologist about any allergies you may have to food or medications. Some anesthetic drugs contain the same proteins as certain foods—especially eggs and soy products, which many people are allergic to—and these drugs will cause an allergic reaction in those people.

Also tell the anesthesiologist what medications you're taking. If you don't know all of their names, bring them with you, for these medications can have a profound effect on the success of your operation.

In my own preoperative meetings with patients, I try to learn their medical history and previous unpleasant experiences with anesthesia, so that I can reassure them by letting them know the same thing won't happen again. If someone has had nausea and vomiting in the past, I'll know to pay special attention to prevent this from happening. Some patients tell me they've had trouble waking up after anesthesia, which suggests that these people are sensitive to the anesthetic drugs, alerting me to give lower doses.

What to Ask

The main thing to remember regarding your preoperative consultation is:

- Don't be afraid to ask the anesthesiologist questions.

Remember, anesthesiologists too have families who have operations. I myself had difficulty once contacting another anesthesiologist in a different town who was caring for my mother. I arrived at the hospital there with her and went along when she was seen by a nurse practitioner for a preoperative consultation. I worried that if only the nurse practitioner saw her, the anesthesiologist would not know enough about her medical conditions, so I asked for the anesthesiologist and was told he'd be in the next morning; no one else was available.

The next morning, when my mother was scheduled for surgery, I was there to talk to him. Our communication was strained, to say the least, because there was not really enough time to fully discuss her problems. In the end, her operation was successful, but I certainly had my share of anxiety waiting for her to arrive in the recovery room. Even anesthesiologists are not immune from anxiety over surgery.

The following general questions apply to any anesthetic procedure.

- Who will be present during my anesthesia? Is that person an anesthesiologist or a nurse specialized in anesthesia?

The type of anesthesia provider you need depends on the procedure you're having and your medical condition. For a complex procedure, such as lobectomy (partial removal of a lung), you'd certainly want an anesthesiologist, preferably board-certified, or at least board-eligible. If, on the other hand, you're a basically healthy person having an inguinal (groin) hernia repaired, a nurse anesthetist is perfectly competent to provide anesthesia, as long as an anesthesiologist is readily available to medically direct your care.

- Will you be present or readily available throughout my procedure—including in the recovery room?
- If this is a specialized operation for a child, ask: Is there an anesthesiologist with specialized training or experience in pediatric anesthesia?
- For cardiac and neurological surgery: Is there an anesthesiologist with specialized training or experience in that subspecialty?
- If I need intensive care, are there critical care physicians present around the clock in the ICU?
- How can I expect to feel after anesthesia? Will I have a sore throat from the endotracheal tube? How soon will the IV lines or special monitors be removed so I can be more comfortable?
- What should my level of activity be right after the operation?
- What treatments are available for postoperative pain?

Most hospitals provide patient-controlled analgesia and epidural analgesia. Some hospitals may not use these techniques routinely—again, because they require extra time on the part of the nurses and the anesthesiologist, who may not feel adequately compensated under the flat-fee arrangement. You may not be offered these techniques, which is why it's so important to discuss them and clearly state what you expect.

Postoperative pain relief is critical for recovery—since when you're in pain, you don't get up and start walking—which is why it's crucial to focus on this subject during the preoperative consultation. Effective pain control is worth fighting for. But you need to know in advance what's available, so you can demand it.

Often a health maintenance organization (HMO) will agree to refer, say, eight patients to an anesthesiologist, paying $200 for each surgical anesthesia but for nothing else. The anesthesiologist will take these patients just to get the business, and may or may not have the time to give the postoperative analgesia anyway. Knowing it won't be reimbursed doesn't help either. Suppose your anesthesiologist does want to give you a postoperative nerve block to control pain, but your HMO refuses to pay separately for it. Call the insurance company to insist that it's a medical necessity. Have the anesthesiologist do the same. If the company still refuses, it's up to you to be aggressive and convince the anesthesiologist to provide it.

Another version of this scenario is that, if your insurance company won't pay for the nerve block, a very busy anesthesiologist is less likely to recommend it to you, since she or he won't receive the additional fee. Only if you know beforehand that it exists can you insist that you want it.

If you're unhappy with the answers to any of the questions listed above, or any other aspect of the care as outlined by the anesthesiologist—or if you feel uncomfortable with the anesthesiologist you see—you might want to request another one. If this fails, ask the surgeon to refer you to another hospital. In some cities or towns there's only one hospital, and you don't have a choice. In such a case you simply have to make the best of what's available, as I had to when I saw my mother's anesthesiologist only on the morning of surgery. If more up-to-date pain relief techniques are unavailable, for example, you'll have to have intramuscular narcotics. Even then, you can maximize the benefits by trying to have someone with you who can chase down the nurse and make sure you get the injections on time.

- Be sure to write down the anesthesiologist's answers to your questions. This is quite important, because under stress it's easy to forget the details. You want to have a written record to refer to later, especially if you wind up seeing different specialists who have different opinions.

Perhaps all this self-advocacy seems too difficult, or just plain exhausting, especially given that needing medical care by definition means that you're not at your best. If you find yourself unable to manage it—whether because you're too sick or because being assertive is difficult for you—perhaps a family member or friend can be your advocate.

Finally, if you feel you've been prevented from getting necessary care, you can appeal to the consumer protection section of your state health department. Should this measure prove ineffective, you can go directly to your state attorney general's office.

Choosing an Insurance Company

In most cases, the best insurance plan is fee-for-service (indemnity), in which the insurance company pays a fee to the provider for every treatment you receive. Since this type of plan is now quite expensive, few can afford it; most people have to consider other options. Only 8 percent of the patients who receive anesthesia in my hospital have fee-for-service plans. Forty percent are in managed care plans, 30 percent are Medicare patients, and about 15 percent get Medicaid. Five percent have private union plans (another form of insurance that's becoming as rare as the dodo bird) or workers' compensation or are self-pay patients—people who have no insurance and are responsible for their own medical bills.

Managed Care Plans

In looking for the best managed care plan, one important indicator to consider is whether the physicians and other members of a plan are happy with it; this is usually a sign of fairness in treatment and in reimbursement to the physician. Doctors usually belong to many plans; ask those you're already going to which are the better ones. Also ask family and friends—especially those who have had surgery—about their managed care companies. Many people have been in numerous plans, since employers have to provide several options.

Next, carefully scrutinize the coverage each plan provides. Do they have bundled carve-out arrangements of the type I described earlier? If so, you may not get good care, for when you have complications the hospital receives no additional fee for treating them. Suppose, after an open-heart procedure, you develop a wound infection and need to return to the operating room to have it drained and treated. Normally, the surgeon would get another fee for this, but not in a carve-out plan. The result could be a delay in treatment, and you can be harmed if the infection gets worse while you're waiting. Here again is a situation that requires you to be aggressive in understanding your coverage and demanding care. Some plans do provide additional fees for complications, so if you can, pick one that does.

Capitated Plans

In a capitated plan, unlike a managed care plan, a single health care delivery system has an agreement with the insurance company to provide all your medical care for a set fee per month. The insurance company pays the fee whether you require treatment or not, and when you go in, the plan must provide all the care you need. (The term "capitated," from the Latin word for head, means per capita, or by the head.) The provider could be a hospital or clinic; frequently, the hospital has a practice building where its physicians have their offices, as well as a pharmacy. The physicians refer you to other physicians in that system for tests and surgery, and your drugs may be supplied by the pharmacy.

Treatment in a capitated system is even more likely to be compromised than in an HMO, since by its nature the system creates still greater pressure to provide minimal care. So my advice is: don't be in a capitated system if you can avoid it.

The Larger Picture

All these types of plans may be offered by employers, and they are also available as individual plans. Employer and group plans are often less expensive, since greater volume allows the insurance companies to charge lower premiums. As more and more people become part-time, temporary, or contingent workers who receive no benefits, the insurance situation is likely to grow increasingly grim.

Nor will it improve, in my opinion, until all Americans have a basic health insurance plan. Since health care is now one of the biggest for-profit sectors in the American economy, insurance companies spend millions of dollars each year to lobby Congress to prevent such a plan from being enacted. Yet it could easily be financed by a minimal tax of 2 to 4 percent on all Americans—following the model of Australia, to pick one example we would do well to emulate. Nor need this insurance be provided by the federal government; the government could contract it out to the existing insurance companies.

Unfortunately, the current system is not likely to change until little profit is left for investors in the health care industry—a development I believe is inevitable. At that point, the large companies will fold, and we will have to create a new system—hopefully, one based not on stock market profit but on ensuring quality health care for every American citizen.

Until that time, you can only improve your prospects by being proactive—asking questions, making demands, and negotiating as best you can to get what you need at every level of the health care system.

Summary: Questions and Points to Remember

- Ask to see an anesthesiologist prior to surgery if your surgery will be complicated—or simply because you want to.

- Be sure to prepare questions about *anything* that is making you anxious.
- Don't be afraid to ask the anesthesiologist questions.

Ask:

- Who will be present during my anesthesia? Is that person an anesthesiologist or a nurse specialized in anesthesia?
- Will you be present or readily available throughout my procedure—including in the recovery room?
- If this is a specialized operation for a child, ask: Is there an anesthesiologist with specialized training or experience in pediatric anesthesia?
- For cardiac and neurological surgery: Is there an anesthesiologist with specialized training or experience in that subspecialty?
- If I need intensive care, are there critical care physicians present around the clock in the ICU?
- How can I expect to feel after anesthesia? Will I have a sore throat from the endotracheal tube? How soon will the IV lines or special monitors be removed so I can be more comfortable?
- What should my level of activity be right after the operation?
- What treatments are available for postoperative pain?
- Be sure to write down the anesthesiologist's answers to your questions. This is quite important, because under stress it's easy to forget the details. You want to have a written record to refer to later, especially if you wind up seeing different specialists who have different opinions.

• • •

Tobacco, Alcohol, Recreational Drugs—and Other Substances— Can Be Deadly

• • •

Linda, a thirty-two-year-old pregnant woman, arrived at our hospital for her second cesarean delivery. When I took her history and examined her, she seemed relatively healthy. But when she came into the operating room, we noticed that both her heart rate and blood pressure were extremely high—which was not the case when I had seen her. Assuming that this reaction was due to presurgery anxiety, I administered a sedative through the intravenous catheter to reduce the anxiety.

But Linda's heart rate and blood pressure only increased. Thinking that inducing anesthesia would relieve this condition, I did so—and these signs rose still further. In fact, her blood pressure was so high we feared that either a blood vessel in her brain would rupture (resulting in stroke), or she'd have a heart attack. I had to give her labetalol to slow her heart and nitroprusside to decrease her blood pressure. These drugs would not have been required had she merely been anxious.

During the early part of the operation I tried several times to discontinue the drugs but could not, for without them Linda's heart rate and blood pressure shot up again. Fortunately, the baby was born without any problems, and I was finally able to stop the drugs during Linda's recovery period. Once she awakened, we asked her if she had previously had hypertension (high blood pressure) and tachycardia (rapid heartbeat). No, she said, she hadn't. What she did have, it turned out, was a habit. She was a crack user. She had brought crack cocaine with her, and just before going to the operating room, she felt anxious, so she took some.

No one had asked Linda, "Do you use any recreational drugs?" during her preoperative interview. Some anesthesiologists would likely be reluctant to ask such a question, for fear of insulting the patient—or it might not even occur to them. And, like most people who use recreational drugs—including alcohol—Linda was not about to volunteer that information. Even if they were asked, some patients might lie, fearing disclosure and possible arrest. Linda was just lucky that we were able to prevent a major complication caused by the interaction between the cocaine she had taken and the anesthetic drugs. Meanwhile, now that we knew Linda had used crack, the delivery unit nurses watched her baby carefully for evidence of cocaine withdrawal, which could have been life-threatening.

Not only illegal drugs but alcohol, tobacco, and even some herbs are potentially dangerous if you use them before having anesthesia. And if you have a caffeine habit, telling the anesthesiologist about it can prevent a wicked postoperative headache.

Alcohol

The hazards alcohol poses for anesthesia and surgery depend on whether patients are actively drunk just before, during, and after surgery or whether they are long-term alcohol users—and also on how much they drink.

When someone has consumed alcohol just prior to surgery, his or her need for anesthesia decreases, and the risk of developing low blood pressure is greater. Alcohol causes hypotension in two ways. First, it dilates blood vessels; and second, it is a diuretic, which means that blood pressure drops because more fluid is lost in the urine.

Chronic alcoholics also require less anesthesia, though in their case this is partly because their livers have been damaged by cirrhosis and can't metabolize the anesthetic drugs. Since the breakdown and excretion of these drugs from the body is considerably delayed, the effects of anesthesia last much longer. Chronic alcoholics also require less anesthesia due to the effects of alcohol on the nerve receptors responsible for the anesthetic state. By contrast, someone who is not a chronic alcoholic but consumes at least four drinks a day will need more anesthesia, since the alcohol induces the liver to produce enzymes that speed up metabolism.

- If you use alcohol, tell the anesthesiologist how much you habitually drink, and the last time you had a drink. Don't drink anything right before surgery.
- Forty-eight to seventy-two hours after your last drink you may have withdrawal symptoms, possibly including seizures. To avoid this, you will need a sedative drug.

The anesthesiologist should know that you need a sedative to avoid withdrawal symptoms. But in case she or he fails to give you this drug, you should request it.

Tobacco

When chronic smokers come to me for surgery, I encourage them to try to give up tobacco completely for just two weeks, to reverse some of its many harmful effects that impact anesthesia administration. Tobacco stimulates the heart, raises blood pressure, and increases the level of carbon monoxide in the blood. The more carbon monoxide the blood carries, the less oxygen it can transport to the tissues. Insufficiently oxygenated blood is particularly hazardous if a problem with breathing occurs during anesthesia.

Chronic smoking also permanently damages the lungs and the heart. In the lungs it causes emphysema and chronic bronchitis. When the lungs are unable to take in enough oxygen, the pressure in the lung vessels increases, and the heart has difficulty pumping blood through the lungs. The heart then becomes enlarged, while continuing to receive an inadequate supply of oxygen. The result is hypertension and tachycardia. These changes too affect the administration of anesthesia.

Long-time smokers also usually have chronic coughs and chest infections that must be treated before surgery. They frequently develop laryngospasm (a contraction at the back of the throat that closes the windpipe) upon induction of anesthesia, and they have reactive airways—which means the air passages in the lungs react to environmental stimulants like odors or cold by constricting, as in asthma. Smokers often need bronchodilators, drugs that open the airways, to prevent their developing bronchospasm during the operation.

If smokers can make it through a two-week abstention from tobacco, our ability to oxygenate their blood during anesthesia improves considerably, since the amount of carbon monoxide in the blood decreases during these two weeks. The asthmalike wheezing they experience when they're smoking also diminishes, which further improves oxygenation during their surgery.

During this two-week hiatus, the level of nicotine in the blood drops, which allows the condition of the heart to improve, decreasing the need for additional drugs during surgery. This is important, since the drugs we must use to prevent hypertension and tachycardia can interact with the anesthetics, causing wide swings in blood pressure and heart rate that can lead to stroke or heart attack right on the operating table.

Unfortunately, tobacco seems to be one of the most addictive substances around, and most smokers I've encountered can't follow my suggestion.

My advice may be heard but usually isn't heeded, which is why I always prepare for the worst possible complications when I administer anesthesia to smokers. These complications actually occur about 40 percent of the time. Even so, after the operation smokers return to their cigarettes. This addiction is so powerful that even people with cancer of the mouth who require a tracheotomy—insertion of a breathing tube through an incision in their neck—have been known to smoke right through the tube.

Passive Smoking Hurts Children

If you're a smoker, you should also know that children of parents who smoke are at great risk during anesthesia. A 1998 study reported that children exposed to environmental tobacco smoke had more than twice as many respiratory complications before, during, and after surgery as children who did not have such exposure. These effects included laryngospasm, which prevents the anesthesiologist from ventilating the child's lungs; wheezing; bronchospasm, a constriction of the air passages of the lungs, which causes wheezing and severe coughing; and severe coughing when anesthesia was induced or discontinued. The researchers noted that girls were more susceptible to the effects of second-hand smoke than were boys.

In my own experience, children who have been exposed to tobacco smoke often begin to wheeze when anesthesia is administered, making anesthesia management much more difficult. Frequently, we must give the child a bronchodilator, which may increase blood pressure. We use an inhalation anesthetic, which decreases wheezing, but because large amounts of the drug are required, blood pressure may drop.

When we reverse the anesthesia in these children, they are more likely than other children to cough and develop laryngospasm. Because the air passages in the lungs are spastic and likely to contract, these children are also at greater risk of developing pneumonia after surgery. This occurs because the constriction inhibits the normal process of clearing waste matter, including infectious bacteria, from the lungs.

- If you smoke, be careful to avoid doing so in the presence of your children, or at least make sure that ventilation is sufficient to prevent the children from inhaling your second-hand smoke (passive smoking).

Caffeine

Before Marjorie's breast biopsy, her doctor told her to fast, starting at midnight before her 11 A.M. surgery. "I was already feeling caffeine withdrawal before the procedure—shaky, bitchy, headachy—and it got worse as the day wore on," she recalled. "In the recovery room, the first thing I asked for was a cup of coffee." But her headache got worse and worse, until she felt as though "my head was going to blow off." She called her surgeon and talked him into prescribing Valium, which put her to sleep. When she woke the next day, she was fine, but she had gone through hours of utter agony that could have been prevented.

Headache is a common complaint after general anesthesia. In the past, we thought it was a side effect of the anesthetic drugs we used. Recent studies, however, have shown that it is frequently an effect of caffeine withdrawal, since patients are routinely instructed to fast before surgery. It's been estimated that over 80 percent of adults in North America drink coffee and other caffeinated beverages. If people who regularly consume caffeine go without it for as little as eight hours, they begin to develop the withdrawal symptoms that Marjorie described: irritability and headache.

For this reason, some anesthesiologists are now giving caffeine prophylactically, either before surgery or just afterward. Since Marjorie started developing a headache before her surgery, she may have needed caffeine then to prevent her headache from becoming full blown. Patients who are unable to drink after surgery can receive caffeine tablets through a nasogastric tube. Those whose caffeine consumption is high can also be given caffeine intravenously during the operation.

- If you regularly drink caffeinated beverages—even as little as one cup a day—tell your anesthesiologist this and ask for some form of prophylactic caffeine. Or you could simply drink a cup of coffee or tea (without milk) four hours prior to surgery.

Illegal Drugs

Even after years of working in a large inner-city hospital, I'm always surprised at how many of my anesthesia patients use recreational drugs. These patients, by the way, come from every profession and every socioeconomic class; even pilots may be addicted to heroin. Many doctors, too, are seriously addicted to a variety of pain relievers, stimulants, tranquilizers, and muscle relaxants, according to an August 1999 *New York Post* report; the article described one anesthesiologist who was hooked on the high he got from fentanyl. If you take drugs, you have a lot of company, so don't let a sense of shame lead you to keep your drug use secret when you're facing surgery.

Why You Should Admit Drug Use

Experience has taught me always to ask about recreational drugs during the preoperative visit. At first people were reluctant to disclose that they had a habit. But I learned to emphasize that their surviving the operation might depend on my knowing about any drug use, and to assure them that whatever they tell me would be kept confidential. Once they received both the warning and the reassurance, they could admit that they took drugs.

When patients use addictive drugs, we have to continue their habit in order to prevent withdrawal before, during, and after surgery. We do this to save their lives, since suddenly discontinuing their usual drugs could actually kill them. We therefore continue the addiction during this period, either with their own drugs or with similar ones. For example, all narcotics have similar effects on heroin users and will prevent acute withdrawal symptoms. For chronic alcoholics, we use a tranquilizer such as Librium to prevent withdrawal and seizures.

When patients come to see me the week before surgery and admit that they use addictive drugs and if the surgery is not an emergency, I refer them to a drug rehabilitation center. If the surgery is an emergency, I administer similar drugs to prevent withdrawal complications such as extreme anxiety and even seizures. Since I'm controlling what they take, I can control what happens in the operating room. After surgery, we continue giving those drugs or similar ones to prevent withdrawal. When the patients are ready to go home, we recommend a drug treatment center or program in the hope that they'll take advantage of it.

- If you or a family member having surgery uses a recreational drug, overcome your reluctance and tell the anesthesiologist about it. Otherwise, you may literally not survive to take it again.

Cocaine

Cocaine constricts the blood vessels, increasing heart rate, possibly causing life-threatening arrhythmias, and raising blood pressure. Entirely on its own, it can cause heart attacks and congestive heart failure. Cocaine users often have abnormal heartbeats, and administering anesthetics to them may lead to cardiac arrest. Chronic users may develop cerebral aneurysms (pouches formed by the weakened, dilated walls of blood vessels in the brain), which can rupture and bleed during surgery and anesthesia and, if not detected, cause death. Cocaine also damages mucous membranes, leading to abnormalities in the structures of the mouth and nose that can make airway management difficult, such as erosion of the hard palate or of the cartilage that separates the nostrils. Powder cocaine, by the way, has the same effects as crack.

Since cocaine itself is an anesthetic, when a patient has taken it just before surgery, as Linda did, the anesthesiologist can't use the normal dosage of anesthetic drugs. Upon awakening from anesthesia, chronic users may develop seizures that could compromise the airway. Cocaine is one of the most destructive drugs around; thus chronic users are among the most difficult patients to manage for anesthesia.

Marijuana

Marijuana acts on your system like a mid-level anesthetic. It also increases the heart rate and reduces blood pressure. If you smoke marijuana before surgery, your anesthesiologist must reduce the amount of anesthetic drugs you receive. If he or she is unaware of the need to do this, you face serious problems with your heart and blood pressure.

Long-term marijuana use affects the lungs much like long-term tobacco use, causing chronic cough and respiratory impairment. Thus it's important to tell the anesthesiologist if you've smoked a great deal of marijuana in the past, even if not in the period just before your surgery.

Heroin

Heroin has many side effects that affect anesthesia. A major problem we have with heroin addicts is that it's difficult to give them intravenous anesthetics; since they've used all their veins to give themselves fixes, the veins are so scarred that we literally can't find any site where we can insert the needle. Second, as a narcotic, heroin reduces the amount of anesthetic drugs needed when it is taken just prior to surgery. Next, since heroin users are addicts, if they require emergency surgery at a time when they haven't been able to get a fix, they may develop symptoms of withdrawal: seizures, diarrhea, severe anxiety, and general hyperactivity. These patients must receive narcotics as part of anesthetic management, since inhalation anesthetics won't prevent withdrawal symptoms in the postoperative period. Another difficulty is that, because these patients have developed a tolerance for narcotics, they require larger doses of these drugs for pain relief after surgery than do nonaddicts.

If someone has a previous history of heroin abuse but has stopped using the drug, the anesthesiologist must avoid giving that person narcotics in order not to trigger the addiction again. Instead this patient should receive inhalation drugs.

Heroin users have lung problems, since this drug, which is injected, contains impurities that lodge in the blood vessels of the lungs, preventing adequate oxygenation of the blood and making anesthesia more difficult to administer. Heroin users also have abnormal kidney function and are at risk for kidney failure during anesthesia and surgery.

Finally, like all intravenous drug users, heroin addicts have depressed immune function and are at risk for infectious diseases, such as HIV and hepatitis B and C, which have their own effects on anesthetic management. People with hepatitis may have difficulty metabolizing anesthetic drugs, which can worsen their liver infection. Those with HIV have several organs affected, and the anesthesiologist must be aware of possible preexisting nerve, kidney, and liver damage, which might require that lower doses of anesthetic drugs be used.

We can prevent the worst of these effects if we know in advance that the patient is a heroin user; that's why it's essential that drug users not hide their habits from their anesthesiologist.

Special K

Special K, or ketamine, is an anesthetic drug that is stolen from hospitals and pharmacies and used on the street because in small doses it causes vivid hallucinations. Its effects last longer than those of cocaine. Like cocaine, it stimulates heart rate and raises blood pressure, causing the same problems that we see in cocaine users.

Ecstasy

Ecstasy, or MDMA, is an amphetaminelike (stimulant) drug that heightens awareness and may cause hallucinations. There have been reports of fatal seizures and liver damage after its use. Users may take Ecstasy before surgery, thinking it will let them simply float through the experience without being bothered by anything. But in fact it increases their risks. For one thing, it's impossible to get an accurate history or do a complete physical exam of patients who are high on this drug; unable to concentrate or even speak clearly, they can't answer questions. When people take Ecstasy after surgery, it often makes them unable to notice and describe symptoms of any complications that may be developing.

Angel Dust (PCP)

Angel dust (phencyclidine, also known as PCP), which is used by veterinarians to tranquilize large animals, is another popular street drug. Its effects combine those of Ecstasy and cocaine, which means that when it interacts with anesthesia it can raise heart rate and blood pressure dangerously high, while preventing the user from noticing that anything is wrong.

Ethyl Chloride

Ethyl chloride is a liquid anesthetic that is sprayed on the skin; people who use it recreationally pour it on a cloth and sniff it to get high. It can cause irregular heartbeats that are particularly dangerous during anesthesia. Ethyl chloride may also induce liver and kidney toxity, which can alter the effects of anesthetic drugs.

Amyl Nitrite

Amyl nitrite, a drug that dilates blood vessels, is used to treat priapism (abnormal, painful erection) and to prevent erections after circumcision, which would be painful. In contrast to the drugs described above, it has a relaxing effect; the high it induces is partly due to low blood pressure resulting from the dilation of the vessels. People feel light-headed, dizzy, as though they're floating. If amyl nitrite is used before anesthesia and surgery, it can cause severe hypotension.

Herbs

You might not think of herbs as dangerous substances on the order of the illegal drugs described above, or even alcohol and tobacco. But in fact, when combined with anesthesia they can have effects just as serious.

A third of Americans now use herbs such as St. John's wort, *Ginkgo biloba,* and ginseng. And many believe that because herbs are "natural," they aren't "drugs" and are therefore safe. This is why, according to a recent study, seven out of ten patients who take herbs don't tell their doctors about them.

But herbs are actually potent medicines—that's why they work. What's more, if your anesthesiologist doesn't know you're taking them, they can be dangerous, because they can interact with anesthetic drugs or cause bleeding or changes in blood pressure during surgery.

- St. John's wort, taken to relieve anxiety, sleep disorders, and depression, affects blood pressure and can increase the effects of some anesthetics.
- *Ginkgo biloba,* used to boost blood circulation and improve memory, may result in bleeding because it decreases the number of platelets, cells in the blood that are needed for clotting.
- Ginseng, widely taken to promote vitality, may result in hypertension and tachycardia.
- Feverfew, taken to relieve headaches, can also interfere with blood clotting and therefore result in bleeding.
- Ephedra (also called *ma huang*) has been used to treat asthma and upper respiratory infection and is also taken to increase energy and promote weight loss. It appears to cause fluctuations in blood pressure, irregular heartbeat, and other serious reactions.
- Garlic, taken as an immune system booster, inhibits platelet function and can increase bleeding during surgery.

It's wise, therefore, to stop taking herbal medicines at least two weeks before surgery so that they can be cleared from your system. If you don't have two weeks to do this before the surgery is scheduled, bring the herbs in their original bottles to show the anesthesiologist exactly what you're taking. This is important, because herbal products are not regulated by the Food and Drug Administration, and they may include other ingredients aside from the herb named on the label that could affect anesthesia and surgery. If your anesthesiologist and surgeon (who has to control any increased bleeding) know before the operation what herbs you've been taking, they can control any adverse effects.

Summary: Questions and Points to Remember

- If you use alcohol, tell the anesthesiologist how much you habitually drink, and the last time you had a drink. And don't drink anything right before surgery.
- Forty-eight to seventy-two hours after your last drink, you may have withdrawal symptoms, possibly including seizures. To avoid this, you will need a sedative drug.
- If you smoke, be careful to avoid doing so in the presence of your children, or at least make sure that ventilation is sufficient to prevent the children from inhaling your second-hand smoke (passive smoking).
- If you regularly drink caffeinated beverages—even as little as one cup a day—tell your anesthesiologist this and ask for some form of prophylactic caffeine. Or you could simply drink a cup of coffee or tea (without milk) four hours prior to surgery.
- If you or a family member having surgery uses a recreational drug, overcome your reluctance and tell the anesthesiologist about it. Otherwise, you may literally not survive to take it again.

PART 2

Anesthetic Care for Specific Medical Problems

CHAPTER 6

• • •

Childbirth and Women's Health

• • •

"I can honestly say that I felt no pain in preparation for or during the surgery—not from the injection for the epidural, not from anything at all—and so I'm glad I was able to forgo the general anesthetic," wrote English professor Regina Barreca, describing her experience of a hysterectomy for *Sunshine* magazine. "I wanted to be conscious as soon as possible so that I could actually face the experience of what I was going through." She was asleep during much of the procedure, but woke up in time to ask to see her uterus, which the surgeon had just removed, and to joke that when he sewed her up, he should embroider "If You Can Read This, You're Too Close" in an appropriate location.

Barreca's generally positive experience of having a hysterectomy reflects the fact that most hospitals have now made women's health a priority. This new focus—triggered by the women's health movement, which, beginning in the 1970s, changed the medical profession's entire approach to treating women—is partly why infant mortality associated with childbirth has declined since then. Still, not only for pregnancy and childbirth, but also for gynecological procedures, such as Barreca's, and for non-obstetrical procedures performed while you are pregnant, you can get the best care if you know what to ask for, as she did when she requested an epidural.

Pregnancy and Childbirth

Early in my career on an anesthesia rotation, I was assisting at a delivery. "Let me show you how to drop ether," the nurse anesthetist said. At that time, we used an inhaler with a mask; you put the mask over the patient's face and dripped ether on it. In this case, the expectant mother weighed three hundred pounds (which, as I'll explain later, increased her risk under anesthesia) and had eaten just before going into labor. The nurse kept dripping the ether, and the woman breathed in too much of it. She vomited and sucked the vomitus into her lungs, stopped breathing, and began to turn blue. Resuscitating her was extremely difficult, because large chunks of food blocked her airway, and this plus her obesity made it hard to see the opening into her trachea. We managed to revive her, but it was horrendous. I thought, "There's got to be a better way than this!" That experience was one reason I decided to become an anesthesiologist. I wanted to teach people to look for a better way of administering anesthesia—especially to pregnant women.

The Changes of Pregnancy

During pregnancy, a woman's body undergoes anatomical and physiological changes that alter the way anesthetic drugs affect her. These changes are quite normal, but it's important that the mother herself as well as her doctors be aware of them.

Because the growing baby exerts pressure on the lower parts of the mother's lungs, the volume of air her lungs hold decreases. She breathes rapidly and becomes unable to tolerate even short periods of breathlessness. For this reason, a woman in labor should not receive large amounts of sedative drugs, which would depress her respiration even more, to the point where she could not maintain adequate oxygen levels in her blood. This in turn could harm the baby.

Pregnancy also brings increases in the hormone progesterone and in overall metabolism to support the needs of the growing baby, placenta, and uterus. These changes lead in turn to an increase in the heart rate and in the total volume of blood circulating in the body. Another effect of progesterone and of the increasing blood flow to the placenta is to dilate blood vessels, causing a slight decrease in blood pressure. Some sedatives also relax the blood vessels. When used during labor and delivery, they increase the dilation of these vessels normally induced by pregnancy, so the mother could develop low blood pressure and be unable to deliver enough oxygen to the fetus. Since sedative drugs given intravenously pass readily through the placenta, they depress the baby's respiration and blood pressure as well. This is why we try to avoid using sedatives for women in labor.

In pregnancy, the stomach empties more slowly, so it is generally always full. Thus there is a risk of vomiting and aspiration should general anesthesia be required. What's more, the increased levels of progesterone cause a relaxation of the gastric sphincter—the lowest part of the esophagus, which prevents the stomach contents from flowing backward into the esophagus. If the woman begins to vomit during induction of anesthesia, before the breathing tube is placed, aspiration can occur, resulting in severe pneumonitis (lung inflammation) and even death. This is what could have happened to the woman described above.

The combined result of these changes of pregnancy is that women require lower doses of anesthetics during labor and delivery. The increased progesterone decreases the dose of anesthesia needed, while the dilated blood vessels impinge on the space around the spinal cord where the drugs are placed for an epidural. Since there is less space, a normal dose of anesthetic would be pushed farther up the cord and affect higher parts of the body, possibly interfering with breathing and further decreasing blood pressure as the anesthetic causes more blood vessels to lose their tone.

Finally, the position for giving birth also affects anesthetic management. If the mother lies on her back, as is common, the baby presses on the inferior vena cava, the major vein passing up the trunk of the body, and prevents the blood from returning to the heart. The result is low blood pressure and possible harm to the fetus. For this reason, it is better to lie on the side than on the back to give birth. An anesthesiologist who sees a decrease in blood pressure needs to determine whether this is an effect of pressure on the vena cava rather than of the anesthetic. Careful monitoring of a woman in labor can prevent harm to the baby from wide swings in blood pressure and inadequate oxygenation.

Choices for Anesthesia

I recommend regional anesthesia for labor and delivery, since it eliminates the greatest risk of general anesthesia: vomiting and aspiration of stomach contents into the lungs. A regional also allows the mother to be awake during delivery and immediately bond with the baby. In fact, although some women do choose general anesthesia, this is rare. Most have a regional anesthetic.

Some obstetrical anesthesiologists manage labor pain with small doses of narcotics given intravenously or intramuscularly—a far less complex and less expensive way to provide analgesia. The small doses used are safe for both mother and baby; they are so low, however, that they may not control labor pain to the degree the mother might want. To me, giving narcotics during labor seems risky, since these drugs can potentially depress the breathing of both mother and baby—while at the same time not relieving pain adequately. However, I'm not an obstetrical anesthesiologist.

If your doctor offers you this option, remember that it is used safely in this country by experienced specialists.

- If your anesthesiologist offers you intravenous or intramuscular narcotics for labor pain, ask what the benefits are. Then decide for yourself whether you want this form of pain control.

Spinal or Epidural?

If you want analgesia during labor, you need an epidural. With an epidural catheter in place, we can continuously adjust the level of analgesia, balancing the woman's level of pain against her ability to push. Since large doses of local anesthetics may make her less able to push, we generally give small doses, either of a local anesthetic, a narcotic (which provides more pain relief), or a combination of both.

For what's commonly referred to as a "walking epidural," we administer a small dose of narcotic into the spinal canal by means of a spinal needle placed through the epidural needle. (Giving the drug through the spinal needle jump-starts the narcotic; if we simply placed it into the epidural space through the epidural catheter, the onset of analgesia would take at least 15–20 minutes.) The spinal needle is then removed, and an epidural catheter is threaded into the epidural space. The narcotic lasts one to one and a half hours, allowing the woman to walk around during that time. After this dose wears off, we can inject a very dilute solution of local anesthetic mixed with the narcotic. Adding the local makes the analgesia last longer; but if she had a more concentrated dose, we couldn't let her walk, since the local anesthetic could make her legs weak.

Delivery

Delivery is often more painful than labor, because of the stretching of the perineum (the skin around the vagina) that occurs, because many women have an episiotomy (an incision made to enlarge the vaginal opening), and because sometimes a forceps is used, which increases pain. During the last part of pushing, just before delivery, we often give larger doses of local anesthetics, with or without narcotics, injected into the epidural catheter. This catheter is occasionally left in place so we can provide analgesia well into the postpartum period by injecting additional drugs.

Some women—particularly those who have had babies before—have very rapid labors and may not need an epidural catheter. For them, a single injection in the low back of narcotic or local anesthetic as a "saddle block" (which numbs your bottom, the part that sits on a horse) may provide adequate pain relief for both labor and delivery.

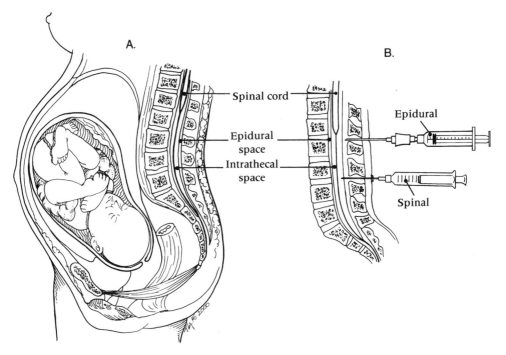

Fig. 7. Administering epidural and spinal anesthesia to a pregnant woman. (A) Anatomy, showing the spinal cord, intrathecal space, and epidural space. (B) Placement of epidural and spinal.

In the past, delivery room staff would give the mother a mask attached to the anesthesia machine or an inhaler consisting of a little canister, so she could breathe an inhalation anesthetic such as nitrous oxide during painful contractions. This is sometimes still done in small community hospitals. But I strongly recommend that you not accept this form of anesthesia unless you're attended by an anesthesiologist trained to monitor your reaction to the drug. Otherwise, because a pregnant woman's ability to tolerate anesthetic drugs is diminished, using an inhalant could lead to unconsciousness, vomiting and aspiration, and death.

Cesarean Delivery

Most cesarean deliveries can be performed under regional anesthesia. A cesarean requires a larger dose of epidural anesthetic than is needed for a vaginal delivery, because there's a lot more pain. We can also give a spinal; if there is still pain, the obstetrician can inject local anesthesia directly into the area where it's felt.

You should not have general anesthesia for a cesarean if it can be avoided. Ask for a regional—it's safer for both mother and baby.

Anesthetic Considerations for Uncomplicated Delivery

Sometimes obstetrical anesthesia is delegated to a nurse anesthetist. In my opinion, this is not an acceptable practice, since the risk of anesthesia for pregnant women is high, and when a problem does occur it's life-threatening for both mother and child. I believe that practitioners with more specialized training should provide anesthesia for labor and delivery—preferably an anesthesiologist specialized in obstetrics, who can not only administer the regional but place monitors and treat any complications. In fact New York, the state where I practice, requires that a facility with a complex obstetrical suite have an anesthesiologist in house twenty-four hours a day, seven days a week, to handle emergencies.

Most often, women about to give birth are seen by the anesthesiologist when they enter the labor and delivery unit. At this time, the anesthesiologist reviews all the information related to the pregnancy and orders lab tests if any are indicated. Having this information beforehand prevents the anesthesiologist from being called in at the last minute without knowing anything about a patient's particular needs. So if you plan to have anesthesia, be sure to request that you see the anesthesiologist.

During this visit you should ask:

- What anesthetics are available? If you prefer a particular anesthetic, be sure to request it.
- Who will be administering my anesthesia? How available will that person be during my labor and delivery?
- If you have chosen natural childbirth, ask whether someone will be available to provide anesthesia should you change your mind during labor or delivery.

Sometimes women who had planned on natural childbirth decide during labor or delivery that the pain is too great and they ask for relief.

Complications

A small but growing number of women choose home birth and do without anesthesia altogether. This is fine, as long as there are no complications. One reason good prenatal care is important is that it enables the obstetrician to predict when a woman is likely to have a complicated delivery requiring qualified anesthesia personnel. Frequently, the obstetrician arranges prenatal clinics at which groups of pregnant women and their partners can ask an obstetrical anesthesiologist questions about anesthetic management for delivery and discuss their options. This practice is fairly common in large regional medical centers, though community hospitals may not offer it.

Often an obstetrician will refer a woman who is likely to have a complicated delivery, or who has a significant medical problem, to the anesthesiologist for an individual appointment in advance, so a management plan can be worked out.

- If your obstetrician anticipates a complication, ask if you can talk with the anesthesiologist before you go into labor. This consultation will not only make you feel more comfortable but will give your child the best opportunity to survive and thrive.

Preeclampsia and Eclampsia

Preeclampsia is a complication of pregnancy involving high blood pressure; sudden swelling of the face, hands, or feet; headache; rapid weight gain; and excess protein in the urine (which is how it's diagnosed). The cause is unknown, but some evidence suggests preeclampsia may be an autoimmune condition in which the mother's body rejects parts of the placenta. Preeclampsia occurs most often in very young pregnant women, usually under fifteen; in those over forty; and in those with preexisting hypertension and diabetes. It also tends to recur, so that a woman who has preeclampsia during her first pregnancy has a higher than normal—though still not very large—chance of developing it in subsequent pregnancies.

If untreated, preeclampsia can develop into eclampsia, a condition that involves life-threatening seizures and coma. So we treat preeclampsia with a combination of antihypertensive drugs and magnesium sulfate, a drug that prevents seizures by stabilizing nerve conduction in the brain.

Among women with preeclampsia and eclampsia, anesthesia for labor and delivery is particularly complicated because of the potential for wide swings in blood pressure. We generally give an epidural because of its tendency to improve uterine blood flow and because it's useful to have a reliable anesthetic in place, since these women are more likely to require a cesarean delivery. Since eclampsia is a medical emergency requiring immediate treatment, there is sometimes no time to place an epidural catheter, and then we must give a spinal.

- If you have preeclampsia, be sure to ask for an epidural, because it improves uterine blood flow and may help prevent increases in blood pressure.

Abnormal Presentation

When the baby is positioned abnormally in the birth canal—as, for example, in a breech presentation, where the buttocks or feet are facing the opening of the uterus—the anesthetic plan may be changed. We may perform a regional anesthetic, spinal or epidural, and relax the uterus with intravenous nitroglycerin to make delivery easier. Rarely, these measures are insufficient to deliver the baby, and a general anesthetic may be necessary. Here we would use an inhalation anesthetic, which also relaxes the uterus.

Sometimes delivery is still not possible, and we must perform a cesarean. The uterine relaxation caused by the inhalation drug will result in increased bleeding after the delivery, so we stop the inhalation anesthetic as soon as the baby is delivered. This enables the uterus to regain its tone and the bleeding to stop before the surgeon closes the mother's abdomen. We switch to an intravenous anesthetic to control pain while the surgeon closes the uterus and abdominal wall.

Multiple Births

Multiple births are not exactly a complication, but they do require a change in the anesthetic plan similar to that for abnormal presentations. Often it's necessary to relax the uterus in order to position the second baby for delivery. Thus if the mother started out with a regional, we may need to give her nitroglycerin or even general anesthesia, which we do after placing an endotracheal tube. In some cases of multiple births, the anesthesiologist may decide to give general anesthesia from the beginning.

- If you have a breech presentation or will be having multiple births, ask whether the anesthesiologist will be available should you need to switch from regional to general anesthesia.

Often the anesthesiologist will place the epidural and then leave the patient in the nurse's hands. But if a switch is required, you need the anesthesiologist there.

Other Conditions That Complicate Childbirth

A number of common conditions can complicate anesthesia for childbirth.

Diabetes. Diabetics usually have larger babies because their abnormal metabolism delivers extra quantities of glucose to the developing fetus. Thus diabetic women are prone to cephalopelvic disproportion, which means that the baby is too large to move down the birth canal and must be born by cesarean.

During labor and delivery, we must closely monitor a diabetic mother's blood sugar levels. Blood sugar that is too low could cause brain abnormalities in the fetus. The anesthesiologist raises blood sugar by administering a solution containing a form of glucose called dextrose. On the other hand, high blood sugar has a diuretic effect that could result in low blood pressure if too much fluid is excreted. High blood sugar is also associated with sudden fetal death during the pregnancy. The need for tight control of blood sugar may mean that even women who are not strictly insulin-dependent must take insulin while they are pregnant.

- If you are diabetic, ask that your blood sugar levels be monitored at frequent intervals during pregnancy, labor, and delivery.

Obesity. Obesity creates a number of problems for anesthesia in pregnant women. Obese women frequently have high blood pressure and are at greater risk for aspiration, abnormal breathing, and inadequate oxygenation. The dose of anesthetic drug they receive must be very carefully adjusted. Preferably, an obese woman should have an epidural, but the catheter is more difficult to place because there is so much fat around the spine.

If we can't place the epidural, we can attempt a spinal. If we can't give that, we must give general anesthesia, which is quite risky in obese patients because aspiration and hypertension can occur during induction.

- If you are overweight, stress to the anesthesiologist that you prefer regional anesthesia.

Asthma. Asthma is another difficult problem requiring careful management. A pregnant asthmatic must comply rigorously with her current drug regimen. If her asthma worsens during labor and delivery, inadequate oxygenation of her blood will jeopardize the baby. Since stress can trigger an attack, analgesia during labor and delivery is highly recommended for asthmatics. To avoid emotional upset as well as physical stress, we might place the epidural earlier than usual, at the very beginning of labor, then adjust the dosage so the mother can continue to push during contractions, but without any pain.

- If you're asthmatic, be sure you comply with your treatment plan. Notify your anesthesiologist if you're wheezing or if the medications aren't controlling your asthma.

Valvular Heart Disease. Some pregnant women have a condition that affects the valves of the heart. The most common such conditions are mitral valve prolapse (in which the valve between the two left-hand chambers of the heart never completely closes, so that blood flows when it's not supposed to) and rheumatic heart disease (which causes clogging and hardening of the valves, impairing blood flow).

Valvular abnormalities, on top of the physiologic changes of pregnancy, make anesthesia much more difficult to administer, and women with these conditions are at far greater risk of complications from the anesthetic during labor and delivery. The specific abnormality and valve involved determine which anesthetic technique we use. (For details, see the sections "Special Considerations for Valve Surgery" and "Valve Surgery" in chapter 9.)

- If you have valvular heart disease, ask if the delivery site you've selected can handle patients with your condition.

Usually, you need a regional medical center. Most community hospitals will not have staff who are able to place the necessary monitors or who are familiar with the drugs required to treat the abnormal heart rhythms that occur.

Abnormal Blood-Clotting Conditions. If you have a condition that prevents your blood from clotting normally, you may not be able to have regional anesthesia. Examples of such conditions are Von Willebrand's disease, a genetic deficiency that prevents blood clotting, and idiopathic thrombopenic purpura, a lack of sufficient blood platelets (small cells required for clotting to occur).

- Be sure to notify the anesthesiologist that you have such a condition far in advance, and keep reminding all your care providers about it.

Many of the nonsteroidal anti-inflammatory drugs (NSAIDs), particularly aspirin and ibuprofen, are extremely long-acting. Even a single dose of aspirin can interfere with blood clotting for as long as two weeks. Having an NSAID in your bloodstream might prevent you from having spinal or epidural anesthesia, since there's a chance that you might bleed into the epidural space. The result would be a hematoma, a mass of blood that can compress the spinal cord and cause paraplegia.

- Avoid taking any NSAIDs as the time of your delivery draws near.
- Notify your anesthesiologist if you have recently taken any of these drugs—even an aspirin for a headache.

Abruptio Placentae and Placenta Previa. In abruptio placentae, the placenta becomes detached from the wall of the uterus, causing severe pain, possibly life-threatening bleeding, blood-clotting problems, and premature labor. This condition requires emergency delivery, and general anesthesia is the quickest way to do so; though if blood loss is minimal, it may be possible to use regional anesthesia.

In placenta previa, the placenta covers the opening of the uterus. During labor it separates from the uterine wall, and can cause life-threatening bleeding. Most cases of placenta previa are diagnosed early in pregnancy, however, and a cesarean is scheduled to deliver the baby—often under regional anesthesia—before bleeding occurs.

Nonobstetric Surgery for Pregnant Women

Should you require anesthesia for nonobstetric surgery during your pregnancy, you should know how to avoid these potential hazards: fetal abnormalities, induction of preterm labor, and aspiration caused by the physiologic changes of pregnancy. Women having surgery during pregnancy have a higher incidence of miscarriage, but this may be due just to the stress of surgery itself and may not be related to the anesthetic drugs they receive.[1]

Fetal Abnormalities

Fetal abnormalities related to anesthesia are most likely to occur during the first trimester. Routine use of unnecessary drugs, such as sedatives and antiemetics, should be avoided during this period. Although no evidence confirms that antiemetics (drugs given for nausea and vomiting) are teratogenic (cause physical defects in the fetus), there is also no certainty that they aren't—except for the phenothiazines, which appear to be safe. The drug ondansetron (which is not a phenothiazine) is commonly used intravenously for nausea and vomiting in the operating room, but no evidence demonstrates that it is preferable to the phenothiazines.

- If you need an antiemetic, make sure you get a phenothiazine, such as Phenergan.

During the preoperative consultation, we try to soothe a pregnant woman's anxiety that the surgery will harm the fetus, in order to avoid having to give her sedatives. If that's not possible, we give a barbiturate, such as phenobarbital, instead of a benzodiazepine. This is the only sedative that is safe to use.

- If you're pregnant and having surgery, tell the anesthesiologist that you don't want any unnecessary drugs.

Though inhalation anesthetics administered to pregnant women, as well as surgery itself, may result in a slightly greater risk of miscarriage, clinical studies done with large numbers of patients found no links between these drugs and an increased incidence of congenital anomalies. In all these studies, however, the number of women who were given anesthetics during the first trimester was too small to enable us to conclude that these anesthetics definitely do not harm the fetus in that early period. We prefer to delay surgery to the second trimester if that does not create significant risk to the mother.

Induction of Preterm Labor

No studies have found that anesthetic drugs or techniques create a greater risk that labor will begin prematurely. The location of the surgery does affect the likelihood of preterm labor, for the closer to the uterus the procedure is performed, the more likely it is that labor will be induced.

- Ask that your uterine activity be monitored, especially in the postoperative period, to detect the possible onset of preterm labor, so you can receive treatment immediately to prevent miscarriage.

General Guidelines for Surgery during Pregnancy

- Defer any elective surgery until after delivery and after the physiologic changes of pregnancy have reverted to normal (usually about six weeks).
- If you are of childbearing age, be sure to have a urine pregnancy test before having any surgery.
- Should you need urgent surgery—that is, the procedure is essential but can be delayed somewhat—wait until the second or third trimester.

- If you need emergency surgery that can't be delayed past the first trimester, remember that the best available data suggest that it's safe for the baby. I believe, however, that the best anesthesia to have in such a case is a regional block.
- Since the pregnant uterus can block blood flow in the vena cava if the patient lies on her back, it's important in any type of surgery to make sure a pillow is placed under your right hip, to displace the uterus to the left. Also ask that a fetal heart rate monitor be used, especially after the sixteenth week.

Common Gynecological Procedures

Most of these procedures are performed by an obstetrician/gynecologist.

Hysterectomy

Hysterectomy, or removal of the uterus, is the most frequently performed gynecological procedure. Generally, it is done to remove fibroids (this was why Regina Barreca had hers), as well as in cases of endometriosis (in which tissue that normally lines the inside of the uterus grows outside it in the pelvic cavity), abnormal bleeding due to other causes, and cancer of the uterus. Often a hysterectomy can be performed through the vagina, but if the uterus is too large to remove that way, an incision in the lower abdomen is necessary.

Anesthesia for both abdominal and vaginal hysterectomy is the same: we generally give a regional—most often an epidural. The epidural pro-vides appropriate operating conditions for surgery and, as in other cases, allows for more effective postoperative pain management.

Sometimes, however, we also give general anesthesia for abdominal or vaginal hysterectomy. For a vaginal hysterectomy the patient must lie with her feet in stirrups and her head down. Particularly if she is obese or has large breasts, she may find not only that this position is uncomfortable, but that it interferes with breathing. Such a patient may be more com-fortable having general anesthesia.

Invasive carcinoma of the uterus, with involvement of the surround-ing lymph nodes, requires a radical hysterectomy, with removal of the uterus, ovaries, and nodes. For this procedure we must provide a high level of anesthesia for a long period of time, which often means giving general anesthesia.

- If you're having a vaginal hysterectomy, consider whether you might prefer general anesthesia, and discuss this question with your anesthesiologist before surgery.

After a hysterectomy with general anesthesia, your options for postoperative pain control include all of those described in chapter 2: epidural analgesia, patient-controlled analgesia, or intramuscular narcotics.

Removal of Ovaries

Endometriosis, painful ovarian cysts, and ovarian cancer sometimes require removal of the ovaries. Surgical anesthesia and postoperative pain control for this procedure are essentially the same as for hysterectomy.

Cervical Cancer

Cancer of the cervix, or cervical carcinoma, may involve various stages of surgery. A loop electrocautery excision procedure (LEEP, in which electric current is passed through a wire loop) may be performed for cervical dysplasia (cells that show precancerous changes). Laser vaporization is used to remove cancer in situ (still confined to its original site). With cone biopsy, a cone-shaped tissue sample is removed from the cervix by LEEP, scalpel, or laser.

For these procedures, less analgesia is required than for hysterectomy or ovarian surgery, and we can give mask inhalation anesthesia. Postoperative pain is minimal—or you may need only acetaminophen.

For more invasive surgery, such as resection of the lower part of the cervix, a spinal may be more appropriate and will also help block pain after the procedure. If necessary, we can also give patient-controlled analgesia to relieve postoperative pain.

Minor Gynecological Procedures

Tubal ligation, termination of pregnancy, and dilation and curettage (scraping away of the lining of the uterus) are generally performed under general anesthesia, simply because these procedures are so short; placing a regional would take longer than the procedure itself.

Tubal ligation, a form of sterilization in which the fallopian tubes are "tied" and cut or surgically blocked, is usually done one day after delivery, in order to allow the uterus to return to its normal size. This makes the procedure easier for the obstetrician to perform. (If you have a cesarean, the ligation may be done during that operation.) Since the physiological changes of pregnancy take much longer than one day to return to normal, the anesthesiologist must manage the airway carefully to prevent aspiration.

For termination of pregnancy before sixteen weeks, performed in a hospital, we induce anesthesia with a sedative, then give a short-acting narcotic and small amounts of an inhalation anesthetic. Abortion is also frequently performed in free-standing clinics, where no anesthesiologist may be present. In such a case, conscious sedation or local anesthesia (in which the anesthetic is injected into the cervix) should be available; both options should provide adequate pain control. Since for many women, abortion brings up intense emotional issues, you may also want to request an antianxiety drug.

After sixteen weeks, an abortion is a difficult procedure for the anesthesiologist, since by this point the changes of pregnancy that create the risk of aspiration are present. Placement of an endotracheal tube is absolutely necessary to prevent aspiration. We induce anesthesia with a sedative and give an intravenous narcotic, but no inhalation drug. This combination is usually sufficient, since the procedure is so short. If the patient needs more anesthesia, we give her more of the sedative.

- If you seek an abortion, be sure you know how many weeks pregnant you are. This information can really mean the difference between life and death, for the anesthesiologist needs to know whether the physiological changes of pregnancy are present or not.

Laparoscopic Gynecological Surgery

A laparoscope is a thin telescopelike instrument with a light that is inserted through a small incision in the abdomen. It allows the surgeon to visualize the abdominal cavity for diagnosis and to perform surgery with tiny instruments inserted through additional incisions. Laparoscopic surgery is done to correct infertility and to diagnose abdominal pain, ovarian cysts, and endometriosis. It requires slightly inflating the abdomen with carbon dioxide, which expands the abdominal wall away from the pelvic organs, making it easier to view them.

Unfortunately, this gas is absorbed into the bloodstream, raising the level of carbon dioxide in the blood. The carbon dioxide must be eliminated because it will increase heart rate and raise blood pressure. We do this by inserting a breathing tube and hyperventilating the woman during the procedure so that her lungs will excrete the excess carbon dioxide.

Because of this need to eliminate carbon dioxide by having the anesthesiologist breathe for the patient, we rarely use regional anesthesia for laparoscopic procedures. When we do, it's only for patients who are not hypertensive and don't have abnormal heart rhythms. The surgeon must also be comfortable with the patient having a regional.

- If you had or have cardiac rhythm disturbances or high blood pressure, request a general anesthetic, since a regional will worsen these conditions.

Bladder Surgery

As women age, their pelvic muscles tend to weaken, often after pregnancy and childbirth, and their pelvic tissue may atrophy after menopause. These changes can lead to incontinence, or loss of bladder control. Sometimes the uterus drops into the vagina, pulling the bladder with it or pressing on the bladder, causing urgency and uncontrolled urination.

Although there are nonsurgical treatments for incontinence, these may not work, and women may choose to have one of several surgical procedures that attach the uterus to the muscles at the back of the pelvic wall and/or attach the bladder to the fascia (strong fibrous sheaths around muscles) surrounding the pubic bone. These procedures may be done vaginally, laparoscopically, or through an abdominal incision.

Surgery for incontinence requires the head-down position, so some patients need general anesthesia in order to be comfortable. For younger women who are not overweight, an epidural may be appropriate. But even if you choose a general, you should have a continuous epidural placed for postoperative pain management, since there is considerable pain afterward.

- If you're having bladder surgery, ask for an epidural that can remain in place up to seventy-two hours for postoperative pain relief.

Breast Cancer Surgery

Surgery for breast cancer includes biopsy, lumpectomy, and different forms of mastectomy. Breast biopsy is often performed by general surgeons, since obstetricians and gynecologists are generally not trained in this procedure. Frequently, the lump must first be identified by radiology before the patient goes to the operating room for the biopsy. She receives a shot of local anesthesia so the biopsy needle can be accurately placed under radiologic visualization. Then she is brought into the operating room, where she receives her local anesthesia with conscious sedation or general anesthesia, depending on her preference, so the surgeon can take the biopsy. Certainly the local is safer, but if you choose general anesthesia, ask to have it administered via a mask over your face instead of through an endotracheal tube, to avoid having a sore throat afterward.

To treat breast cancer, some surgeons perform lumpectomies, others do modified radical mastectomies, while still others prefer radical mastectomies. The pros and cons of these procedures are still being debated. As yet, there is no clear evidence that a radical mastectomy is any better than a lumpectomy if the nodes are not involved, or that the reverse is true either.

For a lumpectomy (removal of the lump only), as for a breast biopsy, you can choose between local anesthesia with conscious sedation and general anesthesia. A modified radical mastectomy, in which the breast and lymph nodes in the armpit are removed, always requires general anesthesia because it involves a level of pain that conscious sedation and local anesthesia cannot relieve. In addition, during this procedure pressure is applied to the chest that prevents it from expanding enough for respiration to be adequate, so the anesthesiologist must control the patient's breathing.

Radical mastectomy, in which the pectoral (chest) muscles as well as the breast and lymph nodes are removed, also requires general anesthesia. Since this operation is lengthy and often involves considerable loss of blood, we may also place one or more special monitors: an arterial line to monitor blood pressure, a Foley catheter to monitor urine output, and sometimes a central venous pressure catheter, which is inserted into a major vein to measure the pressure and volume of blood returning to the heart. We mostly use this invasive monitoring when the patient has significant medical problems, such as congestive heart failure.

During a mastectomy, the arm on the side being operated on is stretched out to that side. If it is extended too far, weakness and even paralysis can occur because stretching the nerve decreases its blood supply.

- Ask your anesthesiologist to be careful not to overextend your arm on the side of the surgery.

Facing the prospect of breast surgery, you're coping not only with anxiety related to anesthesia and surgery but with the emotional effects related to distortion or loss of an important part of your body and to having a life-threatening disease. It's important to try to separate the fear of anesthesia and surgery, which in this context are essentially minor concerns, from those other, more profound fears. This will help you optimize your treatment and maximize your chances of getting well.

Summary: Questions and Points to Remember

- If your anesthesiologist offers you intravenous or intramuscular narcotics for labor pain, ask what the benefits are. Then decide for yourself whether you want this form of pain control.

During the preoperative visit you should ask:

- What anesthetics are available?
- Who will be administering my anesthesia? How available will that person be during my labor and delivery?
- If you have chosen natural childbirth, ask whether someone will be available to provide anesthesia should you change your mind during labor or delivery.
- If your obstetrician anticipates a complication, ask if you can talk with the anesthesiologist before you go into labor.
- If you have preeclampsia, be sure to ask for an epidural, because it improves uterine blood flow and may help prevent increases in blood pressure.
- If you have a breech presentation or will be having multiple births, ask whether the anesthesiologist will be available should you need to switch from regional to general anesthesia.
- If you are diabetic, ask that your blood sugar levels be monitored at frequent intervals during pregnancy, labor, and delivery.
- If you are overweight, stress to the anesthesiologist that you want regional anesthesia.
- If you're asthmatic, be sure you comply with your treatment plan. Notify your anesthesiologist if you're wheezing or if the medications aren't controlling your asthma.
- If you have valvular heart disease, ask if the delivery site you've selected can handle patients with your condition.

If you have a condition that prevents your blood from clotting normally:

- Be sure to notify the anesthesiologist of this far in advance, and keep reminding all your care providers about it.

- Avoid taking any NSAIDs as the time of your delivery draws near.
- Notify your anesthesiologist if you have recently taken any of these drugs—even an aspirin for a headache.

If you're pregnant and having surgery:

- If you need an antiemetic, make sure you get a phenothiazine, such as Phenergan.
- Tell the anesthesiologist that you don't want any unnecessary drugs.
- Ask that your uterine activity be monitored, especially in the postoperative period, to detect the possible onset of preterm labor, so you can receive treatment immediately to prevent miscarriage.

General Guidelines for Surgery during Pregnancy

- Defer any elective surgery until after delivery and after the physiologic changes of pregnancy have reverted to normal (usually about six weeks).
- If you are of childbearing age, be sure to have a urine pregnancy test before having any surgery.
- Should you need urgent surgery—that is, the procedure is essential but can be delayed somewhat—wait until the second or third trimester.
- If you need emergency surgery that can't be delayed past the first trimester, remember that the best available data suggest that it's safe for the baby. I believe, however, that the best anesthesia to have in such a case is a regional block.
- Since the pregnant uterus can block blood flow in the vena cava if the patient lies on her back, it's important in any type of surgery to make sure a pillow is placed under your right hip, to displace the uterus to the left. Also ask that a fetal heart rate monitor be used, especially after the sixteenth week.

Guidelines for Common Gynecological Procedures

- If you're having a vaginal hysterectomy, consider whether you might prefer general anesthesia, and discuss this question with your anesthesiologist before surgery.

- If you seek an abortion, be sure you know how many weeks pregnant you are.
- For laparoscopic gynecological surgery, if you had or have cardiac rhythm disturbances or high blood pressure, request a general anesthetic, since a regional will worsen these conditions.
- If you're having bladder surgery, ask for an epidural that can remain in place up to seventy-two hours for postoperative pain relief.
- If you're having a mastectomy, ask your anesthesiologist to be careful not to overextend your arm on the side of the surgery.

NOTE

1. The information in this section is based on Sol M. Shnider and Gershon Levinson, *Anesthesia for Obstetrics*, 3d ed. (Baltimore: Williams & Wilkins, 1993).

CHAPTER 7

• • •

The Extremes of Age: Anesthesia for the Young and the Elderly

• • •

In the past, when anesthesiologists planned anesthesia for children, they thought of them as little adults—except that because young children's nervous systems were not fully developed, they were believed to have less pain perception than adults and no memory of whatever pain they did experience. This belief persisted for many years, and because very young children cannot verbalize the pain they feel, their other ways of responding to it were frequently underrated or even ignored.

When I first trained in anesthesiology, surgery on children, such as circumcision and even hernia repair, was often performed using muscle relaxants to prevent the child from moving and interfering with the surgery—and with very little anesthesia. Even fairly recently, children often received less analgesia than did adults for similar surgical procedures and were much less likely to receive postoperative pain medication.

Now, however, we know that children's ability to handle drugs and fluids is very different from that of adults, and that they require different management to keep their organs functioning under the stress of a surgical procedure. We also know that even the tiniest baby feels pain. Numerous studies have shown that children's pain responses are as intense as those of adults, and we know that observing certain signs in a preverbal child—an increase in heart rate and blood pressure, a strong cry, a particular facial grimace—is the same as hearing an older child scream: "It hurts!" Today, various pain scores allow us to evaluate even preverbal children's levels of pain and the effectiveness of the pain-relieving medications we give them.

We know too that a hospital experience can have a real psychological impact. Recent surveys have refuted the notion that the memory isn't sufficiently developed for the child to have any lasting recollection of it or experience negative consequences later. We've learned that children do remember unpleasant experiences and can have exaggerated reactions even to minor painful situations in later years. And we are acutely aware of the fears and concerns parents have when they entrust their precious children to us.

Today, children commonly receive anesthesia for surgery, as well as conscious sedation for minor procedures such as MRIs (see next section for a description). If your young child needs surgery, try to ensure that the anesthesiologist is a pediatric specialist. If that's not possible, ask for an anesthesiologist who's at least had experience doing anesthesia for children. A child in pain should be treated just like an adult, without fear of overusing anesthetic drugs. At the same time, the anesthesia provider must understand the child's physiological response to drugs, which is quite different from that of adults.

Like children, people older than seventy-five or so have a different physiology from younger adults. The second part of this chapter will describe their special anesthetic requirements.

Children's Physiological Differences

Pediatric anesthesia is a subspecialty that deals primarily with children under two. These children, and to a lesser degree those between two and seven, seem to do better with a highly trained and/or experienced specialist because their physiological differences from adults make anesthesia for them both different and difficult to administer. A child has a very high metabolic rate, which creates a greater need for oxygen. Yet the child's lungs contain a smaller volume of air. Since the lungs have only small oxygen reserves, if breathing stops even briefly, the existing supply of oxygen will be rapidly used up. Thus a child is at much greater risk for respiratory and therefore cardiac arrest under anesthesia.

In addition, children need more anesthesia in proportion to their body weight than do adults, since their higher rate of metabolism means that the anesthetic drugs stay in their system for a shorter time. They also have a higher respiratory rate, which means that anesthesia can be induced more rapidly—and that they emerge from anesthesia more rapidly too.

In one case, a two-year-old being anesthetized for repair of a hernia suddenly developed laryngospasm (contraction of the larynx, or voice box). Within two minutes he developed bradycardia (an abnormally slow heartbeat) and turned blue. If his airway had not been restored instantly, his heart would have stopped. This is just one example of the extra skills required of the pediatric anesthesiologist, who must be able to react far more quickly when an emergency occurs in a child than is necessary with adults.

Children also respond quite differently to drugs. Using the wrong muscle relaxant to treat the two-year-old's laryngospasm, for example, might have worsened his bradycardia and brought on cardiac arrest, which wouldn't have happened with an adult.

Unlike adults, children can't maintain their body temperature during anesthesia. They become hypothermic—that is, their temperature drops significantly—in a normally cold operating room. Hypothermia in turn poses a number of dangers, including bradycardia, impaired blood clotting, and a longer duration of action of anesthetic drugs. For this reason, during surgery on a young child the operating room must be kept at body temperature.

Very young children under anesthesia have difficulty excreting fluids and some electrolytes (substances essential for conduction of nerve impulses; these substances must be kept in a precise balance). Also, their kidneys can't handle the fluids we administer to adults. So we must give these children both different fluids and different amounts of fluids than we give adults.

Premature newborns face still other hazards: first, hyperventilating (breathing too fast) for the infant can cause hemorrhage into the brain tissues from the immature blood vessels. Second, since high concentrations of oxygen are toxic to the retina and can cause blindness, the anesthesiologist must administer a different mixture of gases, to dilute the oxygen to a safe concentration.

A mother brought her child to our hospital for repair of an inguinal (groin) hernia. During the preoperative consultation, she gave the anesthesiologist the child's entire medical history, including the fact that the girl had been premature. The anesthesiologist knew that children born prematurely often develop apnea (stop breathing) after receiving anesthesia if not carefully monitored in the recovery room for at least twelve and up to as many as twenty-four hours. He was therefore able to prevent a life-threatening complication by ordering that this monitoring be done.

As this story indicates, for children the preoperative visit with the anesthesiologist is crucial.

- Be sure to tell the anesthesiologist if your child has had any previous adverse reactions to anesthesia.
- If your child has had an adverse reaction before, request that she or he be scheduled for surgery first thing in the morning.

If your child is the first case of the day, the anesthesiologist will have more time, before the rush of the day begins, to set up the special equipment and drugs that would be needed to handle any complications.

- If the anesthesiologist whom you see for the preoperative consultation is not the same one who will actually be administering your child's anesthesia, ask that the other anesthesiologist be alerted to the potential problems.

Children under Two

Generally, anesthetic considerations are different for children under two years and those over two. Younger children, who can't be reasoned with, require special attention not only from the anesthesiologist but also from the nurses and, of course, the parents.

Be aware that if your child is sick—for example, has a cold, fever, or rash—the surgery will be canceled, since anesthesia is much riskier under these conditions. Parents usually know when their child is sick.

- If you think your child is sick, call the anesthesiologist or surgeon the day before surgery is scheduled to see if it can still be done.

Preoperative Management

Be aware that your child will have to go without food and water for some time before the operation. The purpose here is not to punish the child but to prevent vomiting during induction of anesthesia.

Children recognize the differences between their usual environment and the operating room. To help decrease their anxiety and make the entire procedure as stress-free as possible, parents should remain with their child right up to the moment anesthesia is induced; bringing their favorite toy or blanket sometimes helps decrease their anxiety. I've seen children brought to the operating room screaming and thrashing about in a caged bed—a dreadful ordeal for the child and for the anesthesiologist as well. The tremendous anxiety generated results in the production of large amounts of adrenaline (the hormone associated with the "fight or flight" response), which can lead to a whole slew of problems.

High levels of adrenaline can make induction difficult, while agitation results in coughing due to the large amounts of secretions caused by crying, as well as actual difficulty breathing. The baby's temperature rises, increasing the metabolic rate, which means the child needs more oxygen, which in turn heightens the risk of trouble during induction. The adrenaline response also causes trouble after the surgery. Less able to fight off infections, the child is more likely to develop pneumonia or an infection in the surgical wound.

Contrast that screaming child with another, who's brought to the operating room being comforted while gently held in a mother's or father's arms. We let the mother hold the child even as we administer sedative drugs through the mouth or rectum. In fact, we often ask the mother to help administer these drugs, since she knows her child's reactions. She continues holding the baby as the sedatives do their job. Only then do we carry the child into the operating room proper. Often we let the mother carry the baby in and keep holding him or her as the anesthesiologist places the mask over the child's face to induce general anesthesia. Your child will not be frightened in the operating room if he or she has been sedated and has a favorite toy or blanket to hold. At this point the stress for the child, parents, and anesthesiologist has been avoided, and we ask the parents to leave the operating room.

Anesthesia during Surgery

A combination of sedation and general anesthesia, which avoids the use of needles, is the technique most commonly used for anesthetizing children under two. Almost all children, when faced with a needle, become uncooperative and try to avoid it. That's why, unless there's a contraindication, we induce by inhalation. If there is some reason why induction must be done intravenously—for example, the child has a full stomach—we can manage this too with a minimum of stress by using a local anesthetic in the form of a cream. After the cream has been on the skin for a while under a Band-Aid, we can insert the needle without pain. Here too we can sedate the child through the nose or rectum until the cream starts to work.

- Remember that sedation is a benefit for your child.

Don't be concerned if the child appears drunk before surgery begins; this is just the drug doing its job.

Some physicians have used narcotic patches (described in chapter 2) to calm children. But because the drug used in the patch can arrest breathing, it's critical to watch the patient constantly. If a doctor offers to use this method, be sure someone is present for the duration of the procedure. I personally consider these patches too dangerous to use.

For longer surgeries, soon after the induction with general anesthesia, we place an IV catheter so the anesthesia can be supplemented with narcotics and muscle relaxants. With this catheter in place, if airway complications occur before the endotracheal tube is inserted—which takes a while—we can give intravenous drugs, which work right away, to correct any breathing abnormalities.

For children under two we use special breathing circuits that maintain the right temperature as well as humidity. Using this equipment requires specialized knowledge of potential complications it can cause. For example, under some circumstances the child might breathe in already-exhaled carbon dioxide and develop a rapid heart rate and rise in blood pressure. By observing the monitors, a properly trained anesthesiologist can tell that this is happening and increase the flow of gases to the child.

As a rule, children under two receive general anesthesia, because they can't lie still on the table even for short periods. Sometimes, however, we administer a regional block after inducing general anesthesia, which allows us to give a lower dose of the general anesthetic. The regional remains effective for controlling postoperative pain for varying periods of time.

Postoperative Management

Your child may wake up from surgery disoriented, crying, and thrashing about wildly. This is called "emergence delirium" and may occur when the anesthesia wears off quickly. It lasts about thirty minutes. By holding and reassuring the child, you can reorient her and prevent her from injuring herself.

For these young children, postoperative pain management needs to be planned well in advance. Often—say, for inguinal hernia repair, circumcision, or orchiopexy (surgical fixation in the scrotum of an undescended testicle)—before the child awakens from the general anesthesia, we can place a long-acting regional block that could provide pain relief for as long as twelve hours after surgery. This is extremely helpful, both to make the child easier to manage in the recovery room and to allay the parents' anxiety. If the child emerges from the recovery room in distress, crying and thrashing, the parents naturally are upset and themselves require considerable attention from the anesthesiologist and nurses. By contrast, if the child is clearly comfortable, the parents can hold him and, in the process, lessen the staff's workload.

- If your child is having a circumcision, orchiopexy, or inguinal hernia repair, ask: Can you place a caudal block ("caudal" refers to the bottom of the spine) before he awakens?

Children can be given a block on almost any part of the body, and you should certainly consider it. Once more, however, a specialist is required, for such blocks are more difficult to perform on a tiny body, whose anatomy is a bit different. Since the toxicity of the drug is much greater in a child, the anesthesiologist must know what dose to administer. Another possibility is that the surgeon can inject a long-acting local anesthetic into the area.

Often, after the first twelve hours of pain relief, no further pain medication is necessary. But in other cases, as the block begins to wear off, the child feels some pain. Here we use the pain score system to determine its intensity. We look at the baby's movement and note the strength of the cry, whether there's a withdrawal response, a scrunched-up forehead, and similar indicators that we compare to a standard scale. After this assessment, we decide what drugs to use. Although the pain is not as great at this point as it would have been during the first twelve hours after surgery, the child still needs relief, so we administer carefully adjusted small doses of narcotic, given orally or intramuscularly. The anesthesiologist must take great care not to give too large a dose, since the drug may cause nausea and vomiting and slow breathing in these children. For this reason, the parents should always be there when children receive pain medications.

- Request additional pain medication based on your own knowledge of your child's reactions to pain.

Remember, there is no reason for children to have pain. Stress to the doctor or nurses that you know your own child's reactions to pain. Use your own scale to describe how much pain the child is feeling: "This is the most pain my child has ever had—it's severe, she really needs pain relief." "This is a moderate amount of pain." "I can tell that this is a mild pain for him."

- Don't be afraid to ask for narcotics for your child, but remember that they may cause nausea and vomiting.

Children are like adults in that addiction to narcotics during episodes of acute pain is not a major risk. In fact, it would be more harmful—both physically and psychologically—for your child to be in pain than to receive pain-killing drugs. As I've said, pain makes respiratory and wound infections more likely.

- If your child acts differently—is hard to awaken, sleeps too much, or doesn't respond to you normally—immediately call the doctor or nurse. These changes may indicate that the child still has anesthesia on board and/or has received too large a dose of the painkiller.
- Remember, no matter how careful and attentive you and the hospital staff are, the child will not be happy until he's home.

Children over Two

Anesthesia is less risky for children between two and seven, since the physiologic differences are not as great. Their major organs have matured, so we no longer need to worry about brain hemorrhage or inadequate kidney function. However, since the lung volume is still low and the metabolic rate high, these children can also benefit from a pediatric specialist. By the age of eight, children can be managed like adults, by an anesthesiologist without specialized training.

Preoperative Management

Children over two are easier to reason with and distract with toys and games to ease their anxiety before anesthesia and surgery. With the help of sedation and the local anesthetic cream, we can often place an intravenous needle before inducing anesthesia.

Nevertheless, it may be helpful for parents to remain with their child until general anesthesia is induced. By soothing the child's anxiety, they can make induction easier. For these children we use small breathing circuits that are similar to those used for adults and less likely to cause problems than the special equipment for the under-twos.

Consider a Regional. We can give a regional more easily to children over two. For children over six, in fact, who can cooperate better, a regional might be preferable to general anesthesia. We can give it together with sedation.

- If you feel strongly that your child shouldn't receive general anesthesia, and if the child is mature enough to cooperate, ask the surgeon and anesthesiologist for a regional.

Postoperative Management

Children over two need pain relief just as much as those under two, and for them postoperative pain management is often easier since they can tell you how much it hurts. Often, pain medication is administered according to the child's response to a "faces of feeling" score (see Fig. 8). We

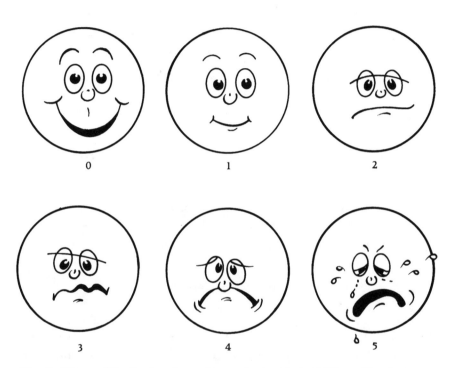

Fig. 8. "Faces of Feeling" scale used to evaluate pain in children. The doctor or nurse explains to the child that each face is for a person who feels happy because he/she has no pain (hurt) or sad because he/she has some or a lot of pain. The child is asked to choose the face that best describes how much pain he/she is feeling.

Face 0 = is very happy because he does not hurt at all
Face 1 = hurts just a little bit
Face 2 = hurts more
Face 3 = hurts even more
Face 4 = hurts a whole lot
Face 5 = hurts as much as you can imagine, although you don't have to be crying to feel this bad

ask the child to point to one of a series of drawings of faces expressing pain that matches how she or he feels. As with younger children, regional blocks administered while the child is still under general anesthesia are critically important to relieve pain immediately after surgery, so the child will feel comfortable in the recovery room and be more able to ward off infections.

Patient-controlled analgesia is also an option, even for children as young as six. We set the pump to prevent overdoses. Still, your presence is essential to assess the effects of the narcotic on your child's level of consciousness as well as on his breathing.

- If your child sleeps too much or seems to be breathing less
  often or less deeply, notify the nurse or doctor immediately.
  Also be alert for hives, which signal an adverse reaction to the
  drug.

It is true that errors can occur in the use of PCA, and overdoses in both children and adults have been reported. That's why your presence is crucial, especially during the initial period after PCA is set up. Sometimes the dosing limit is set too high, so you should be there to note any problems right at the beginning. Still, these problems are extremely infrequent, and the advantages of PCA far outweigh its potential complications.

Commonly Performed Procedures

The surgical procedures most frequently performed on children are removal of adenoids and tonsils, draining of ear infections, hernia repairs, eye surgery for strabismus (cross-eye or walleye), surgery for traumatic injuries (mainly fractures), and correction of congenital anomalies.

Surgery on the head and neck presents particular challenges to the anesthesiologist, since it's hard to keep the windpipe clear. For instance, adenoidectomies and tonsillectomies (removal of adenoids and tonsils) require a smaller than usual endotracheal tube so that the surgeon can work in the same area that the tube passes through. The anesthesiologist must be prepared to deal with possible misplacement of the tube; bleeding at the surgical site, with the chance that blood can run down the windpipe into the lungs; and diminished visibility of the operative site itself.

- If your child has had an adenoidectomy or tonsillectomy, watch
  carefully for bleeding while the child is in the recovery room,

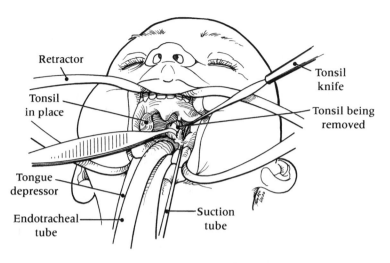

Fig. 9. *Tonsillectomy, showing how the anesthesiologist and otolaryngologist must work in the same small space.*

then at home, and notify or call the nurse or physician if you see any. On rare occasions the child begins to bleed after returning home and must be brought back to the hospital for more surgery.

Children having *eye surgery* frequently develop nausea and vomiting due to disturbance of the cranial nerves.

- If your child is having eye surgery, request that the anesthesiologist use an antiemetic (drug that prevents nausea and vomiting), which may help in this case.

Surgery for *scoliosis* is another fairly common procedure. It involves considerable loss of blood, so you need to prepare in advance to reduce the risk posed by blood transfusions. In a procedure called autologous blood transfusion, blood is taken from the child two weeks before surgery, stored in a blood bank, then used during the operation. During the intervening two weeks, the body replaces the lost blood. You can take two other measures as well to reduce the risks of surgery for scoliosis:

- Request that during surgery the anesthesiologist use a cell saver to collect blood that can be reinfused into the child.
- Ask that spinal cord functioning be monitored during surgery.

Since traction exerted on the spine during the procedure can induce permanent changes in the cord that could result in paralysis, you want to be certain that appropriate monitoring is done to prevent this.

Congenital anomalies raise special concerns for anesthesia. These conditions include hydrocephalus (excess fluid in the brain), meningomyelocele (protrusion of part of the meninges, membranes that sheathe the spinal cord, and the cord itself through a defect in the spine), tracheoesophageal fistula (an abnormal opening between the trachea and esophagus), omphalocele (protrusion of part of the intestine through a defect in the abdominal wall), diaphragmatic hernia (protrusion of abdominal organs upward through a defect in the diaphragm), abnormalities in urine flow, and various heart abnormalities. Surgery for these conditions—and for another condition, intestinal obstruction, which may also be a congenital anomaly—is too complicated to describe in any detail here. However, certain general principles apply to all of these procedures.

- If your child requires complex surgery for a congenital anomaly or for intestinal obstruction, ask if a pediatric anesthesiologist is available. If not, ask about the experience of the anesthesiologist who will be managing your child.

An anesthesiologist who has had only the standard two-month training in pediatric anesthesia is most likely not sufficiently experienced. But if this physician has already handled a number of such cases before, he or she probably is competent.

One important concern with children who have congenital anomalies is that they might develop an allergy to latex. This happens fairly often, since these children are repeatedly exposed to the latex in surgical gloves and in other surgical equipment they come into contact with during the numerous procedures required to correct their condition. Reactions to latex range from a minor rash to a full-blown anaphylactic attack (allergic reaction in which severe hypotension and cardiac arrest can occur). Needless to say, the anesthesiologist must be alert to this possibility and prepared to treat all types of reactions. When operating on a child known to have a latex allergy, the entire operating room staff must use special equipment and gloves that contain no latex.

- If your child has had an allergic reaction to latex, it's crucial that you tell everyone involved in the child's care—from the anesthesiologist to the hospital aides—not to use gloves or other equipment containing latex.

- In any case, insist on speaking to the anesthesiologist about the details of the operation.

Diagnostic procedures, such as MRIs, present especially difficult challenges for the anesthesiologist, since sedating children requires extremely precise calculation of the dose. The dangers are illustrated by the incident I recounted in chapter 2, in which an eight-year-old boy nearly died when he was sedated for an MRI. Children are sensitive to sedatives and may be further compromised by their medical condition. When given sedatives, they may develop respiratory depression and it's harder to resuscitate them.

For these reasons, if your child will be receiving conscious sedation, the potential for serious complications is such that you really need a pediatric anesthesiologist. If a specialist isn't available, ask if the anesthesiologist has had experience providing this type of sedation to children. If the answer is no, perhaps you should consider going elsewhere.

General Questions for All Procedures

- Ask if you can remain with your child until he is calm or general anesthesia is induced.
- Ask if you can be with your child in the recovery room as soon as she arrives from the operating room.
- What kind of postoperative pain relief will you provide?
- What signs should I watch for that may indicate problems after surgery?
- Is my child a candidate for regional anesthesia during surgery, or for a regional given for postoperative pain relief?
- Can I help when you administer sedation? Can I hold my child while you induce general anesthesia?

In the past, we were reluctant to let parents into the operating room because of potential complications, such as obstruction of the airway during induction. We were afraid they would interpret any problems as lack of competence on our part. With the newer anesthetics, though, this rarely occurs, and when it does we simply ask the parents to leave until we get it under control. We do ask them to leave once the child is asleep, since many people faint at the sight of their child's blood, and the last thing we need is parents falling down in the operating room and hitting their heads. Besides, if we already have some anxiety of our own about the case, it's intensified when the parents are there to witness the possibility of our being human.

Anesthetic Requirements of the Elderly

Misperceptions exist about pain in elderly people that are similar to those about children. Not only do physicians frequently take it for granted that pain is an inevitable aspect of aging, but some continue to believe an old fallacy that people's ability to feel pain decreases with age. This may be why nursing home staffs often simply sedate patients who scream rather than treating their pain.

"Research shows that older people do feel pain as intensely as younger ones, but they are less likely to seek relief," Stephen Harkins, professor of gerontology, psychiatry, and psychology at the Medical College of Richmond, told *Modern Maturity* magazine. "So an older patient in pain shouldn't just accept his or her condition, but should seek a responsive doctor. Pain and aging don't have to go hand in hand."

One effect of the aging process is that people come to need less anesthesia, since they grow more sensitive to the drugs we use. They also respond differently to postoperative pain-relieving techniques. After about age seventy-five, respiratory capacity significantly decreases, which means there is less reserve available when breathing problems occur. Most other organs also function at lower capacity, with decreased reserves.

When there is pain, for example, the heart might be unable to increase its rate to accommodate the stress, as a younger heart could; instead it becomes ischemic (lacking adequate oxygenation of its tissues). Because the kidneys no longer excrete urine in adequate amounts, the body retains fluid, which can lead to congestive heart failure. Since the liver metabolizes anesthetic drugs more slowly, they remain in the body longer, so we must give smaller doses. The brain has fewer neurons, or nerve cells, so it requires less anesthesia. And the brain circuitry is very delicate, which means that long after the drugs have passed out of the system, some people may experience disorientation, short attention span, and fluctuations in mood or level of consciousness. A small number may suffer confusion, personality changes, and problems with memory.

In addition to the normal changes that occur with aging, elderly people who need surgery often have other diseases that complicate anesthesia. Arteriosclerosis of the heart and blood vessels causes diminished heart function, usually accompanied by high blood pressure. Emphysema or chronic bronchitis further decreases the ability to breathe, making it harder for the anesthesiologist to manage respiration during surgery.

The first important consideration, then, is to carefully evaluate elderly patients preoperatively so as to devise an anesthetic plan that will enable them to survive the surgery. Knowing that someone has diminished heart function, we can prevent wide swings in blood pressure that could lead to stroke. Since these shifts happen quite rapidly, we frequently use an arterial line to monitor blood gases and blood pressure and an electrocardiogram with five electrodes so that we can precisely adjust the doses of anesthetic drugs as the operation proceeds.

A preoperative consultation in which the anesthesiologist learns the patient's complete medical history is crucial to ensure a successful operation.

- Have someone accompany an elderly patient to see the anesthesiologist.

Often, anxiety makes these patients forget important aspects of their medical history. A friend or family member can prompt the patient to recall past problems with anesthesia and surgery and ensure that the anesthesiologist gets a complete list of medications the patient is taking. It's particularly important with elderly people to write down everything the anesthesiologist says because afterward you can give them these notes, which help them remember.

- Ask the anesthesiologist: Do you have experience with elderly patients?
- Have someone stay with the patient immediately before surgery and especially in the recovery room.

A reassuring presence before surgery will help allay anxiety. Even more important, simply by being present in the recovery room and continually communicating with the patient, you may prevent memory loss, disorientation, and anxiety that retard recovery. Pay particular attention to how well the patient breathes, responds to instructions, and urinates, and to her mental status. Does she know where she is, what day it is, and so on? People are often confused, so you need to say: "It's four o'clock. I'm your daughter." Keep repeating the time, date, and place to get the person back to the present.

- Ask when the patient can start being active.

Find out when he can sit up on the side of the bed dangling his feet, and when he can start walking. The faster he can return to normal, the better his mental status will be.

I once managed anesthesia for an eighty-year-old woman having a hysterectomy and repair of bladder prolapse (downward displacement). Not only did I have to contend with the normal effects of aging, but she was overweight and had a serious heart condition. She had been brought by her son from another state, where she had been deemed too sick for surgery. He felt she could be more successfully managed in his own hospital, where he could be near her.

The difficulty was that no matter what we did, there was a risk of her having a heart attack or a stroke during surgery. Despite a careful choice of anesthetic, she developed low blood pressure during induction, so we administered a drug to increase the output of her heart. This raised her blood pressure, and the surgery proceeded, but soon the pressure grew too high. The monitors showed that her heart was becoming ischemic, so we gave her nitroglycerin to reduce the pressure—but then it got too low, so we had to add a vasopressor to raise it again.

We got through the operation, and she was taken to the recovery room, where her heart continued to be ischemic; in fact, she developed a heart attack, which fortunately we were able to treat successfully. She also became somewhat disoriented and confused. But with her family, doctors, and nurses diligently talking to her, correcting her misperceptions, and orienting her as to date and place, she recovered her normal state of mind and eventually went home in reasonable shape. Her case exemplifies how complicated it can be to manage anesthesia for an elderly person with multiple coexisting medical conditions.

Since long-term confusion has sometimes been associated with general anesthesia, it's often best to give an elderly patient a regional. Anesthesia causes confusion because it disrupts the normal brain circuits, perhaps by shunting the neurotransmitters (chemicals that transmit impulses between neurons) to another, unfamiliar path. Since in the elderly the brain has fewer neurons and neural transmission is slower, the additional disruption provoked by the anesthesia may be enough to push people over the edge permanently. Often—particularly after complex operations like heart valve replacement or coronary bypass—we hear, "Why is Uncle Joe different than he was?" Whether such mental changes occur depends on the patient's condition; they're more likely in people with diseased blood vessels.

Although regional anesthesia is preferable theoretically, it's often difficult to give to elderly patients, since, if they are confused to begin with, they won't tolerate lying on the operating table for long periods. On the other hand, using conscious sedation can readily trigger respiratory depression, since these patients have a lower tolerance for drugs.

This leaves us between a rock and a hard place: a regional is better for the patient, but in a long procedure like a hip replacement (which takes four to six hours), people become very uncomfortable and need sedation. Yet when we try to sedate them, they may suddenly stop breathing, so we have to give them general anesthesia and place an endotracheal tube—which leaves us right at the place we wanted to avoid when we decided to give the regional in the first place.

- Ask whether regional anesthesia is available, and if it would be a good choice for this patient. Why or why not?

Summary: Questions and Points to Remember for Children

- Be sure to tell the anesthesiologist if your child has had any previous adverse reactions to anesthesia.
- If your child has had an adverse reaction before, request that she or he be scheduled for surgery first thing in the morning.
- If the anesthesiologist whom you see for the preoperative consultation is not the same one who will actually be administering your child's anesthesia, ask that the other anesthesiologist be alerted to the potential problems.
- Ask if you can remain with your child until he is calm or general anesthesia is induced.
- Ask if you can be with your child in the recovery room as soon as she arrives from the operating room.
- What kind of postoperative pain relief will you provide?
- What signs should I watch for that may indicate problems after surgery?
- Is my child a candidate for regional anesthesia during surgery, or for a regional given for postoperative pain relief?
- Can I help when you administer sedation? Can I hold my child while you induce general anesthesia?
- If your child has had an adenoidectomy or tonsillectomy, watch

carefully for bleeding while the child is in the recovery room, then at home, and notify or call the nurse or physician if you see any.

- If your child is having eye surgery, request that the anesthesiologist use an antiemetic (drug that prevents nausea and vomiting), which may help in this case.

For surgery for scoliosis:

- Request that during surgery the anesthesiologist use a cell saver to collect blood that can be reinfused into the child.
- Ask that spinal cord functioning be monitored during surgery.

For surgery for a congenital anomaly or for intestinal obstruction:

- If your child requires complex surgery, ask if a pediatric anesthesiologist is available. If not, ask about the experience of the anesthesiologist who will be managing your child.
- If your child has had an allergic reaction to latex, it's crucial that you tell everyone involved in the child's care—from the anesthesiologist to the hospital aides—not to use gloves or other equipment containing latex.
- In any case, insist on speaking to the anesthesiologist about the details of the operation.

Specific Guidelines for Children under Two

- If you think your child is sick, call the anesthesiologist or surgeon the day before surgery is scheduled to see if it can still be done.

Remember that sedation is a benefit for your child.

- If your child is having a circumcision, orchiopexy, or inguinal hernia repair, ask: Can you place a caudal block ("caudal" refers to the bottom of the spine) before he awakens?
- Request additional pain medication based on your own knowledge of your child's reactions to pain.
- Don't be afraid to ask for narcotics for your child, but remember that they may cause nausea and vomiting.
- If your child acts differently—is hard to awaken, sleeps too much, or doesn't respond to you normally—immediately call the doctor or nurse.

- Remember, no matter how careful and attentive you and the hospital staff are, the child will not be happy until he's home.

Specific Guidelines for Children over Two

- If you feel strongly that your child shouldn't receive general anesthesia, and if the child is mature enough to cooperate, ask the surgeon and anesthesiologist for a regional.
- If your child sleeps too much or seems to be breathing less often or less deeply, notify the nurse or doctor immediately. Also be alert for hives, which signal an adverse reaction to the drug.

Questions and Points to Remember for the Elderly

- Have someone accompany an elderly patient to see the anesthesiologist.
- Ask the anesthesiologist: Do you have experience with elderly patients?
- Have someone stay with the patient immediately before surgery and especially in the recovery room.
- Ask when the patient can start being active.
- Ask whether regional anesthesia is available, and if it would be a good choice for this patient. Why or why not?

CHAPTER 8

• • •

Brain and Spinal Cord Surgery

• • •

In February 1997 Pamela Harriman, the American ambassador to France, suffered a massive stroke while swimming in the pool of the Ritz-Carlton Hotel in Paris. Hotel staff called the French equivalent of 911, and the emergency medical transport team that responded took her to the nearest hospital, where she died the same day. It was later found that an aneurysm on her right internal carotid artery (which brings blood to the brain) had ruptured, and damage to her brain was too great to be treated. Had this damage been less severe, she could have been transferred to a stroke center, a specialized hospital unit designed to treat stroke patients.

At such a center, a critical care specialist (who could have been an anesthesiologist) would immediately have managed Harriman's airway, controlled her blood pressure, perhaps reduced her body temperature, administered a calcium channel blocker and possibly thiopental, and then taken her to radiology for a definitive diagnosis. This specialist would have continued to support her vital signs until the tests were finished. After the diagnosis, she could have been taken to the operating room, where an emergency craniotomy and clipping of the ruptured aneurysm would have been performed. These measures might have enabled her to survive— though possibly with paralysis on her left side requiring vigorous rehabilitation.

At the close of the 1990s—declared the "decade of the brain" by the National Institutes of Health—we could look back on considerable progress in preventing and treating brain abnormalities. One accomplishment was the development of stroke centers in most major cities. Another was popularizing the term "brain attack," thus beginning the process of educating people to recognize the symptoms of stroke and know what to do when it occurs as readily as they now do for heart attacks. In spinal cord surgery, too, there were great advances. And the decade also saw the further development of neuroradiology, a field that uses radiology for both diagnosis and treatment of neurological diseases.

Brain Surgery

We perform surgery on the brain to prevent and treat strokes and to re-move tumors. But the most common reason for brain surgery in the United States today is head injury.

Head Injury

Head injury is currently the number one killer of young adults (mostly men), and the largest single cause of head injury is motor vehicle accidents. Those who survive an accident and are brought to the hospital frequently need surgery to control bleeding within the cranium (skull). Uncontrolled bleeding leads to the formation of a mass of blood called a hematoma, which presses on the brain tissue adjacent to it, cutting off the flow of blood, and consequently the oxygen supply, to that area of the brain. Adding to this pressure is swelling of the brain tissue itself as an inflam-matory response to injury, further compromising the oxygen supply. After four minutes without oxygen, brain tissue dies and can't be resuscitated. The sooner we can operate, the greater the patient's chance of surviving without major neurological impairment.

When a trauma patient is brought to the emergency room, therefore, we must make a rapid diagnosis by radiology. Generally the patient is taken for a CAT scan to determine the extent and location of any hemato-mas. Often the anesthesiologist sees the patient first in the emergency room, to assess whether the patient's breathing is impaired. If it is, the anesthesiologist places an endotracheal tube to minimize any injury to the brain that may result from lack of oxygen. (See the section below on spi-nal cord trauma for a description of the delicate art of inserting the tube in someone who has or may have a neck or spinal cord injury.) If the anesthesiologist does place the tube, he or she frequently accompanies the patient for the radiological work-up; then, as soon as the diagnosis is made, the anesthesiologist goes with the patient into the operating room for surgery.

Here, the anesthesiologist places an arterial line, a central venous pres-sure catheter (inserted in a vein usually at the base of the neck, to mea-sure the pressure and volume of blood returning to the heart), and a Foley catheter to monitor urine output, since it's essential to monitor fluid vol-ume and rapidly replace any that is lost.

For the surgery, we use anesthetic drugs, usually thiopental, and other techniques to relax the brain and prevent further swelling. "Relaxing" the brain means slowing down its metabolism so that it needs less oxygen and blood flow decreases. We also administer diuretics to dehydrate the brain. The result of these measures is that the brain loses fluid volume, becomes smaller, and falls away from the cranium, making the surgeon's job easier. Meanwhile, it's critical to monitor the patient's blood electrolytes (substances required for conduction of nerve impulses), since strong diuretics may cause electrolyte imbalances.

- Since surgery for head injury takes quite a long time, you should not worry if a family member remains in the operating room for eight to ten hours.

After the surgery, we can place an intracranial pressure monitor, which detects increases in pressure that might compromise blood flow to the brain. The brain can take a long time to recover, so head-injured patients may remain for up to two weeks in the intensive care unit, where we closely monitor their vital signs.

Stroke

A stroke, or brain attack, is the result of a sudden interruption in the blood flow to the brain. One cause of stroke is occlusion of a cerebral blood vessel, as by a clot. This blockage may cause blindness, inability to speak or write (expressive aphasia), paralysis or partial paralysis of an arm or a leg, or other symptoms, depending on which area of the brain is affected.

The second major cause of stroke is rupture of a blood vessel and resulting hemorrhage, as happened to Pamela Harriman. Rupture may be caused by an aneurysm (a pouch formed in the weakened, dilated wall of the vessel), usually associated with chronic hypertension and/or smoking, or by a congenital anomaly known as arteriovenous malformations (see description below). Symptoms are generally the same as for occlusion of a vessel, except that the person also has an extremely severe headache.

Anyone experiencing these symptoms should get to a hospital as soon as possible, preferably one with a stroke center. Time is of the essence, since most of the treatments for stroke must be administered within four hours to minimize the neurological impairment that might result.

Both blood vessel occlusion and hemorrhage due to aneurysm can be treated surgically. The procedures most often performed to prevent and treat stroke are carotid endarterectomy, ligation and/or occlusion of aneurysms on major cerebral vessels, and ligation of feeding vessels to arteriovenous malformations.

Carotid Endarterectomy

If you have arteriosclerosis of the carotid arteries (in which the walls of these arteries, which supply the brain, become hardened and lined with fatty deposits, narrowing the open space inside the vessel), you may experience what are known as transient ischemic attacks, or TIAs. The term "ischemic" refers to decreased blood supply, and a temporary interruption of blood flow to the brain causes strokelike symptoms: blindness or weakness of an arm or a leg that lasts from a few minutes up to twenty-four hours. You must not ignore these symptoms, for they indicate that sometime soon, if the carotid arteries are not opened up, you may have a full-fledged stroke and wind up with permanent blindness or paralysis of an arm or a leg, or both.

Once a physician confirms that you have had a transient ischemic attack, it must be treated with blood thinners to prevent a major stroke. Sometimes too a "clot buster" (a drug with anticoagulant effects) is injected to dissolve the clot. Calcium-channel-blocking drugs, like nimodipine, have been given to dilate the small blood vessels in the area of the brain that may be developing ischemia and thus decrease the likelihood of stroke following a TIA; however, many physicians disapprove of using nimodipine in such a case.

To prevent stroke caused by narrowing of the carotid arteries, a carotid endarterectomy is performed. In this procedure the surgeon makes an incision into the neck, then opens up these vessels and cleans out the fatty deposits that clog them. For details of the anesthetic considerations for this procedure, see the section "Carotid Endarterectomy" in chapter 9.

Clipping of Aneurysms

Cerebral aneurysms are caused by congenital weaknesses in the walls of cerebral blood vessels, which over time develop areas of dilation. People who have had high blood pressure for a long time develop similar outpouchings at the branching points of cerebral vessels, where turbulent flow occurs. Aneurysms are usually graded on a scale of 0 to 5, with 5 being the most severe; severity depends on both size and neurological symptoms.

Patients who have intracranial bleeding due to rupture of an aneurysm in a major blood vessel generally complain of the worst headache they've ever had in their life. This symptom alerts the physician that rapid intervention is necessary. These patients often have severely elevated blood pressure and may also have paralysis of the face, an arm, and/or a leg.

Large aneurysms that have not ruptured may also cause symptoms by exerting pressure on adjacent brain tissue.

As soon as the diagnosis is made, the patient can be started on nimodipine, which prevents vasospasm (spasm of a blood vessel) from occurring when there's been hemorrhage from an aneurysm. Sometimes immediate surgery can be performed, especially when the surgeon and anesthesiologist are skilled at operating on people with this condition. Otherwise the patient is sedated, assigned to bed rest, and monitored for at least a week before having surgery. This delay makes for easier operating conditions, since during this time the brain starts to repair itself and swelling decreases. However, the delay in surgery may increase the risk of a later episode of bleeding into the brain. For grade 0 to 2 aneurysms, the outcome is better if the operation is performed immediately; for the more severe grades, early surgery is less likely to improve the patient's chances of recovery.

Surgery involves opening the bony skull in the area over the affected blood vessel, carefully separating the dura from the brain tissue, then exposing the aneurysm and clipping the vessel in such a manner that the flow of blood through it is not impaired. Since the surgeon uses saws to cut through the bone, the patient is subjected to considerable pressure and pulling. The surgeon uses a microscope, taking great care not to injure the brain tissue adjacent to the aneurysm and to avoid causing the aneurysm to rupture and bleed more. Meanwhile the anesthesiologist must ensure that the patient does not move and that the brain is relaxed.

For this procedure, we choose mostly intravenous anesthetics. Before inducing anesthesia, we give midazolam to help prevent memory of the operation. I myself use a continuous infusion of a barbiturate, a short-acting narcotic, low-dose isoflurane, and a long-acting muscle relaxant. This combination also achieves the critical objective of keeping the patient relaxed and not anxious, so that blood pressure remains well controlled. Since an increase in blood pressure might worsen the bleeding from the aneurysm, we monitor it closely and increase the drug dose if the pressure rises.

Once anesthesia is induced, the surgeon or anesthesiologist places a catheter in the patient's back to drain off cerebrospinal fluid during the operation; this also helps the brain relax and fall away from the blood vessel being operated on. Another measure taken to minimize brain injury is cooling the body; the temperature is reduced between two and three degrees, with the heart monitored continuously for evidence of possible ischemia induced by the cold. Although this technique has not been definitely proven beneficial, many anesthesiologists use it.

To closely monitor cerebral function and blood pressure, we may use an evoked potential monitor or electroencephalography (EEG). Once the aneurysm has been clipped, it may be necessary to increase blood flow with fluids or with vasopressors, drugs that increase the force with which the heart beats the blood out. As we raise the blood pressure in this way, we can actually see a symptom such as arm paralysis gradually resolve.

With all aneurysms, there's a risk of vasospasm, which can cause stroke both during and after the procedure. During surgery, we try to prevent spasm-induced stroke by infusing a great quantity of fluids, until the heart almost goes into failure. The fluid forces the vessels open, allowing blood to flow to critically injured parts of the brain. The anesthesiologist must calculate with great exactness the amount of fluid to infuse in order to give as much as possible without causing heart failure. We use a pulmonary artery catheter to monitor and maintain this balance; it's left in place for twenty-four to forty-eight hours after the surgery.

We may also use a laser Doppler flow probe postoperatively to aid in detecting developing vasospasm. After the surgeon has clipped the aneurysm, this probe is placed directly into the brain just past the injured area to continuously monitor the velocity of the red blood cells flowing through the vessels, which indicates whether the cerebral blood flow is sufficient in that part of the brain.

Arteriovenous Malformations

Arteriovenous malformations (AVMs) are congenital blood vessel abnormalities. Extra arteries, called feeders, grow in the brain and feed directly into veins, increasing the pressure in the veins, which distend and become masses that cause symptoms as they press into adjacent brain tissue. Over time, additional feeders develop and symptoms worsen. Since the walls of the veins are much thinner than arterial walls, eventually they weaken and begin to bleed, causing symptoms similar to those of a ruptured aneurysm. AVMs may also develop after a head injury.

Surgery consists of tying off or occluding the feeders to prevent the involved veins from swelling and rupturing. AVMs are more difficult to manage than aneurysms because of the great care required to identify arteries that can be occluded without harm because they don't supply important parts of the brain. Even so, the patient may subsequently experience changes in personality and emotional outlook. Unfortunately, these are effects that aren't routinely tested for.

Operations on AVMs can last anywhere from six to twelve hours and require the same anesthetic management, with the same special monitors, as do ligations of aneurysms. Here again we choose drugs that make the brain fall away from the blood vessel in question, providing better visualization for the neurosurgeon. This surgery may need to be repeated until all the abnormal vessels have been eliminated. A two-month interval between operations is necessary to allow the brain to adapt to changes in blood flow.

Recovery Period

Postoperative pain control is important for stroke patients, since anxiety may contribute to vasospasm. However, we must also be careful not to administer so much narcotic or sedative as to depress breathing, since a decrease in breathing could be life-threatening. Fortunately, pain after intracranial procedures is only moderate, since there are pain fibers in the dura but not in the brain itself.

- The family of a recovering stroke patient should be alert for decreasing levels of consciousness. Note whether the patient is sleeping too much, has jerky hand or arm movements (which could indicate seizure), arms or legs that seem weak or paralyzed, or a mouth that droops at either edge.

Brain Tumors

When a forty-six-year-old man came to my hospital as a same-day-admit patient to have a tumor on his pituitary gland removed, he saw an anesthesiologist who wasn't specialized in neurosurgery for his preoperative consultation. Although I was the one who actually managed his anesthesia, I saw him only briefly in the operating room before putting him to sleep, and when I asked if he had any questions, he said no.

The surgery went well; although the patient was hypertensive, we were able to control his blood pressure. At the end of the procedure, the surgeons were concerned that as anesthesia was reversed, he might buck and cough on the endotracheal tube, resulting in bleeding from the surgical site or leakage of cerebrospinal fluid through his nose. So I reversed the anesthesia slowly, without pulling his jaw forward (a stimulus we commonly use to hasten awakening), and gave him IV lidocaine (an anesthetic) to keep him from coughing. Once it seemed he could breathe, I removed

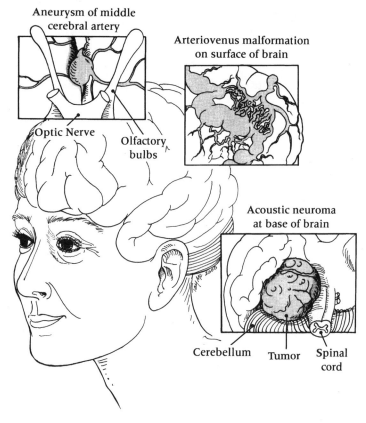

Fig. 10. *Common neurological abnormalities, with their locations in the brain.*

the endotracheal tube. But although he made tremendous efforts, he apparently could not breathe.

Then I noticed that, although his nose was packed from the surgery, he was holding his mouth closed. I told him to breathe through his mouth, but he was still too far under; he couldn't understand me and kept trying to breathe through his nose—until at last he got it, opened his mouth, and was all right. When I saw him the next day, he told me that that moment had been really frightening. But I, assuming he'd been instructed about what to expect, hadn't thought to warn him to breathe through his mouth.

Having surgery on your brain is hard enough without going through a scare like this. Even if you come in as a same-day-admit patient, try to form some kind of relationship with your anesthesiologist so that both of you get the information you need.

Brain tumors occur either in the upper (cerebral cortex) or lower (cerebellum) part of the brain. Tumors in the cerebral cortex cause symptoms largely by increasing intracranial pressure, which diminishes the blood supply, and/or by compressing particular areas of the cortex, such as those that coordinate movement. Once such symptoms occur, we can reduce them by giving the patient steroids, but surgery is necessary to eliminate them.

Preoperative Consultation

Since the anesthesiologist needs thorough knowledge of the tumor's size and location, be sure to bring your records from the neurosurgeon identifying the location of the tumor to your preoperative consultation. This information helps the anesthesiologist decide which monitors to use. We also need to know whether you've had headaches, nausea and vomiting, or other symptoms of elevated intracranial pressure. This will help us determine whether to give you sedatives before the operation.

If you've been put on steroids to reduce the size of the tumor and help maintain blood flow to the brain, tell the anesthesiologist about it. Discontinuing these medications can lead to cardiovascular collapse during the operation, so we have to give them intravenously. Similarly, tell the anesthesiologist if you've been taking diuretics to reduce pressure in your brain. If you have, we need to do blood tests to see whether they've caused any electrolyte imbalances, such as low potassium. If potassium is low, you'll need supplementation.

- When you see your anesthesiologist, make sure you bring your records indicating the size and location of the tumor, symptoms you've experienced, and any medications you're taking.
- If you've had symptoms of elevated intracranial pressure—for example, a severe headache or nausea and vomiting, try not to take sedatives unless you feel you absolutely must.

Surgery for Brain Tumors

During surgery, the anesthesiologist must control the intracranial pressure (that inside the cranium). As a tumor grows, it displaces brain tissue, cerebrospinal fluid, and eventually blood from the cranium. We attempt to restore the blood flow to the affected parts of the brain and to prevent any further interruptions of the flow. To do this we closely monitor blood pressure with an arterial line and urine output with a Foley catheter.

Depending on the size of the tumor, we may use electrophysiologic monitors: EEG or evoked potentials.

To relax the brain, we give the same anesthetic drugs as are used for aneurysms, as well as diuretics. We also hyperventilate the patient to reduce carbon dioxide and constrict the cranial blood vessels. After the surgery, we observe the patient carefully for decreased levels of consciousness, which can indicate bleeding into the surgical site or brain swelling.

Tumors in the cerebellum are more difficult to operate on because they are adjacent to the cranial nerves, which control vital functions, such as heart rate, blood pressure, breathing, and swallowing. Touching these nerves can stimulate abnormal heart rhythms or high blood pressure. Should the surgeon hit a nerve and cause either of these complications, the anesthesiologist must be able to manage it.

Surgery on tumors in a part of the cerebellum referred to as the posterior fossa, which include acoustic neuromas (tumors on the acoustic nerve, the nerve of hearing), is particularly complex. This procedure is sometimes done with the patient's head higher than the heart, and when this is the case, blood moving through veins in the bones that the surgeon saws through may suck in air. This venous air embolism, as it is called, can travel through the blood to the heart and then the lung, where it decreases oxygenation. It may also enter the brain and cause stroke. Before surgery, therefore, we place a Doppler probe on the chest, which detects this air acoustically by means of changing patterns of blood flow into the heart. When the probe diagnoses an embolism, we use the central venous pressure catheter to treat it by aspirating the air from the heart.

Pituitary Tumors

Tumors on the pituitary gland—which, strictly speaking, are not actually within the brain—present major challenges for the anesthesiologist. For example, some secrete a hormone that causes hypertension and obesity in the trunk of the body. Others secrete growth hormone, causing enlargement of the jawbone and tongue, which can make it difficult to place the endotracheal tube.

The anesthesiologist approaches these patients with extreme caution, for in order to remove these tumors, the surgeon must cut open the mucous membranes under the upper lip and go through the nose to expose the cavity that contains the tumor. This is a tricky procedure, which requires that the anesthesiologist have a complete medical assessment of the patient beforehand.

For example, if you have high blood pressure, it must be tightly controlled before surgery, since the surgeon will apply cocaine or another vasoconstrictor to the mucous membranes. The vasoconstrictor decreases bleeding and makes it easier to approach the tumor. But if this drug is used for someone who has had hypertension, the blood pressure can shoot way up, and without rapid treatment the patient may suffer a stroke or heart attack. (See chapter 5 for a description of the effects of cocaine on the cardiovascular system.)

Some pituitary tumors cause massive urine production. Therefore we must place a central venous pressure catheter to signal us to administer large amounts of fluid in case this occurs.

Postoperatively, the anesthesiologist has further problems to address. First, the patient's nose is packed, interfering with breathing, so the anesthesiologist must observe the airway closely. Second, bleeding may occur at the surgical site and block the airway completely. Third, since the pituitary has been removed, the hormones it normally produces will be absent and must be supplemented. For example, lack of antidiuretic hormone may result in diabetes insipidus, a disorder that results in production of excess urine and severe dehydration. Administering vasopressin immediately after surgery will correct this condition but can lead to hypertension, which the anesthesiologist must also be prepared to treat.

- After surgery, observe the urine bag attached to the Foley catheter. If it fills up rapidly, notify the nurse.

Spinal Cord Surgery

We perform spinal cord surgery in cases of injury, to remove tumors, and to correct congenital abnormalities of the spine.

Spinal Cord Injury

Spinal cord injury commonly occurs in auto accidents, but less frequently than head injury; between 20 and 30 percent of head injuries are associated with spinal cord injury. Even the possibility of spinal cord injury requires that the neck be immobilized immediately, since any movement could further compress the cord and cause permanent paralysis.

For the anesthesiologist, this necessity presents a real test in trying to keep the airway clear, since placing the endotracheal tube is difficult when the neck can't be moved. Often we extend the head to make it easier to see the vocal cords, which sit at the opening of the windpipe, but if there's a chance of spinal cord injury, we can't do that. At the same time, these patients' breathing is often impaired due to their injuries; not only must we place the tube without being able to see where it's going, but we have to do it quickly.

Usually, we accomplish this with a fiberoptic laryngoscope, a flexible tube with glass or plastic fibers running through it and a light at the end that projects an image onto a video screen, which shows us where the tube is going. The endotracheal tube itself is threaded over the laryngoscope. Most often the injured patient has a full stomach and therefore must be awake during this procedure, to prevent vomiting and aspiration of stom-

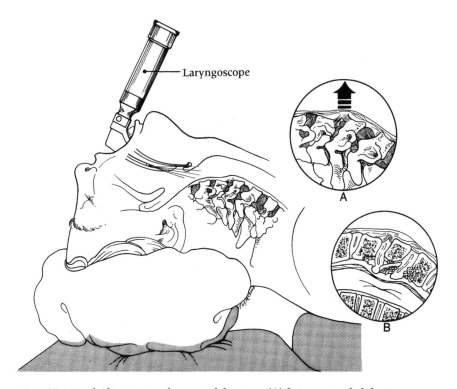

Fig. 11. Head of patient with cervical fracture (A) being extended during airway management. During insertion of the laryngoscope (which is needed for endotracheal intubation), the head may be tilted backward, pushing bone fragments into the cord (B). This poses a risk of paralysis.

ach contents into the lungs. The anesthesiologist, therefore, must first administer a local anesthetic block in the upper airway to eliminate the gag reflex. Once the tube is in position, the patient is asked to move the arms and legs to make sure that the cord wasn't further injured during intubation. It is only then that an intravenous anesthetic can be given that will put the patient to sleep. As soon as this is done, the anesthesiologist begins continuous monitoring with evoked potentials to detect any deterioration of spinal cord function that might be induced.

Spinal Cord Tumors

Tumors of the spinal cord are less common than those of the brain, but they are no less threatening and must be treated quickly to avoid paralysis. Surgery requires that the patients lie face down, which makes airway management difficult since this position prevents easy access. What's more, breathing may be impaired because the patient is lying on his chest and the surgeons may be resting their arms on his back during the procedure. We use an arterial line, a Foley catheter, and evoked potentials to detect early loss of spinal cord function.

As with brain tumors, the anesthesiologist needs to relax the spinal cord tissue and decrease the pressure on it, which we do by using intravenous anesthetic drugs. To ensure amnesia, we may add small amounts of an inhalation anesthetic.

Congenital Anomalies of the Spinal Cord

We often perform surgery to correct two congenital abnormalities: Arnold-Chiari malformation and syringomyelia.

Arnold-Chiari Malformation

In this condition, the back of the skull is too small to hold the brain, so the lower part of the brain is forced down into the spinal canal. The resulting compression of this part of the brain, which contains the cranial nerves, can cause a range of symptoms, including severe pain, headache, abnormal heartbeats and eye movements, sleep apnea (brief cessation of respiration during sleep), and swallowing problems. The degree and nature of the malformation varies; symptoms range from mild to severe, and sometimes the condition is not even detected. Surgery may be done at different ages, depending on how severe the symptoms are. They sometimes worsen with age, as gravity causes more and more brain tissue to drop into the spinal canal.

To correct Arnold-Chiari malformation, the surgeon opens the lower back part of the skull, which allows the brain to return to its proper location. The skull is then closed with a piece of plastic polymer to create additional space. Anesthesia for this procedure is complex, not only because there's a risk of forcing even more brain tissue down the spinal canal—which could cause parts of the brain to die—but because the patient is lying face down, making the airway difficult to manage. We use the same special monitors described above for brain and spinal cord tumors, and choose anesthetics that by relaxing the brain help prevent it from protruding further into the spinal canal.

Since the respiratory centers in the brain may be affected by the surgery, postoperative care focuses on preventing apnea. Often patients stay in the recovery room for at least twelve hours so we can observe their respiration. Since the gag reflex may also be impaired, we don't let patients drink anything for at least twelve hours, to prevent aspiration. It's also possible that a hematoma or swelling will develop in the spinal cord, exerting pressure that results in arm or leg weakness.

- If you are with the patient during this period, watch for signs of coughing or choking, which may indicate aspiration.
- Observe the patient's breathing, especially how strong the breaths are. If you think there's a problem that suggests apnea, call the nurse.
- The patient should be conscious and able to move both arms and legs. If you notice weakness, call the nurse.

Syringomyelia

This congenital anomaly, often present together with Arnold-Chiari malformation, is marked by abnormal cavities in the spinal cord that are filled with cerebrospinal fluid. Syringomyelia often causes severe pain because the dilation compresses the nerve roots (the roots of the major nerves at the point where they emerge from the spinal cord), and patients may be addicted to the narcotics they've been taking to relieve it.

Syringomyelia can develop as a person ages, with the symptoms misdiagnosed until later in life. Surgical treatment is like that for Arnold-Chiari malformation: opening the back of the skull to allow the fluid to flow back into the brain. The surgeon may also place shunts (plastic tubes) to direct cerebrospinal fluid from one section of the spinal cord to another or into the head. These measures all relieve the pressure on the cord and, thereby, the patient's symptoms.

Anesthesia for surgery to correct syringomyelia is difficult for the same reasons as for Arnold-Chiari malformation, plus the possible need to prevent withdrawal symptoms during surgery if the patient is addicted to narcotics. We use the same special monitors as for Arnold-Chiari malformation, and we choose anesthetics that relax the spinal cord in the same way as we relax the brain.

- Tell the anesthesiologist about the symptoms you've been having, and all the medications you've been taking to relieve them—especially to relieve pain.

Neuroradiology

Increasingly, radiology is used not only to diagnose neurological conditions but also as part of treatment. In this case it's referred to as interventional neuroradiology.

Diagnostic Procedures

We perform neuroradiological diagnosis by CAT scan (computerized axial tomography, which produces a cross-sectional view of a selected plane using a series of scans taken at minute intervals, then synthesized into an image by a computer) and by MRI (magnetic resonance imaging, which uses magnetic fields, radio waves, and atomic nuclei to produce detailed cross-sectional images). Both of these procedures require that the patient lie quite still inside a long tube, since any movement will ruin the image. Since the tube makes many people feel claustrophobic, they need sedation, which must be tailored individually to each patient's condition.

For example, sedating someone who has an intracranial mass can be extremely dangerous, especially for children. Sedation depresses respiration and causes increases in carbon dioxide in the blood and consequently in the blood flow to the brain. This further raises the intracranial pressure, leading to possibly catastrophic results: herniation of part of the brain into the spinal canal and cessation of breathing.

For children, the anesthesiologist does a careful assessment beforehand. If we decide that, given mild sedation, the child will be able to cooperate, we do the procedure that way. But if the child seems uncooperative, many anesthesiologists will actually induce general anesthesia in order to be on the safe side, since by placing an endotracheal tube they can control the child's breathing.

Adults may be willing to cooperate, but they often become anxious and start moving around inside the tube. So we give them anxiety-relieving drugs. The danger here is possible depression of respiration and loss of the gag reflex, with vomiting and aspiration. Adults with intracranial masses are also at risk of raised intracranial pressure and herniation of the brain into the spinal canal. Again, the anesthesiologist must calculate the anesthetic dose with precision.

Sedation for these procedures may be done by a nurse anesthetist. This is quite safe, as long as an anesthesiologist is readily available in case a problem arises.

- Ask: Who will manage my anesthesia? Will an anesthesiologist be available throughout the procedure?

MRIs use magnetic fields so powerful that no equipment made of metal can be used near the scanner, for it would be sucked into the tube and possibly injure or even kill the patient. Unless special nonmetallic equipment is available, the anesthesia machine and resuscitation equipment must be kept outside the room, with extra long tubes to reach the patient. The anesthesiologist remains outside and observes the patient through a window.

- Don't bring any metallic objects or credit cards (the magnetic fields will wipe them out) into the MRI room.

A third neurodiagnostic procedure is the angiogram, used to evaluate narrowing of the carotid arteries in stroke patients. Anesthesia for this procedure is described in the section "Carotid Endarterectomy" in chapter 9.

Interventional Procedures

Today, the blood vessel abnormalities that cause stroke are increasingly being treated by a neuroradiologist instead of by a surgeon. For example, we can now thread a catheter through the carotid arteries to the point at which blood flow to the brain is occluded, then either inject a drug that dissolves clots or inflate a tiny balloon to dilate a narrowed vessel; this procedure is called angioplasty. The neuroradiologist performs all the procedures described below using a fluoroscope that shows the vessel and the catheter moving through it on a video screen.

Many of these procedures are done under conscious sedation. The anesthesiologist must calculate precisely the dose of sedative that will keep the patient sedated but still responsive, for the neuroradiologist will need to ask the patient to move the right hand, right foot, eyes, and so on, to test how the procedure is affecting specific areas of the brain.

Neuroradiology can also treat aneurysms and arteriovenous malformations (AVMs), especially when the lesion is located in an area where surgery is difficult or too risky. For an AVM, the neuroradiologist threads a catheter into the feeding arteries and occludes them by injecting a kind of glue. As with conventional surgery for AVMs, the procedure may be done in stages until all the feeding arteries are occluded. This means the patient will have anesthesia several times.

Here again, the patient must be sedated yet alert enough to respond to questions and neurologic exams. If the answers indicate that a neurologic deficit has developed, it's the anesthesiologist who copes. Suppose the radiologist injects the glue into a certain feeder, and the patient then cannot move the left hand. This indicates that ischemia has developed in that part of the brain, perhaps as a result of some glue getting into an adjacent blood vessel or causing a temporary vasospasm. To increase the blood flow in that area, the anesthesiologist increases the blood pressure. Usually, this works, and the patient can move the hand. Sometimes it doesn't, which means the patient has had a small stroke, and function may or may not return.

Occasionally, a major catastrophe occurs: for example, some glue occludes a major vessel and the patient can't move, becomes unconscious, and stops breathing. The anesthesiologist must perform a full resuscitation to restore breathing and possibly take other measures as well to protect the brain.

Certain aneurysms that are either inaccessible by surgery or so large that surgery is too hazardous can be treated by neuroradiology. Here again, the neuroradiologist threads a catheter into the area of the aneurysm and occludes the artery, which decreases pressure in the aneurysm and thereby avoids rupture. To ensure that the artery doesn't feed an important part of the brain, we test the patient's response. Should we find that it's not possible to occlude that artery, another technique is available. If the sac formed by the aneurysm is large enough, the neuroradiologist places a coil resembling an IUD within the aneurysm. The blood clots around it, preventing it from rupturing. Anesthesia for aneurysms is the same as for AVMs except that coiling (placing the coil) requires general anesthesia.

- Since it's important that you remain alert enough to respond to any developing symptoms of ischemia, you may have to experience some discomfort during neuroradiological treatment of an AVM and some aneurysms.

The most painful part of the procedure occurs when the surgeon actually inserts the glue or coil into the aneurysm. This feels like a burning in your head; it's not unbearable pain, just uncomfortable.

Summary: Questions and Points to Remember

- Since surgery for head injury takes quite a long time, you should not worry if a family member remains in the operating room for eight to ten hours.
- The family of a recovering stroke patient should be alert for decreasing levels of consciousness. Note whether the patient is sleeping too much, has jerky hand or arm movements (which could indicate seizure), arms or legs that seem weak or paralyzed, or a mouth that droops at either edge.

For brain tumors:

- When you see your anesthesiologist, make sure you bring your records indicating the size and location of the tumor, symptoms you've experienced, and any medications you're taking.
- If you've had symptoms of elevated intracranial pressure (for example, a severe headache), try not to take sedatives unless you feel you absolutely must.
- After surgery, observe the urine bag attached to the Foley catheter. If it fills up rapidly, notify the nurse.

For surgery for Arnold-Chiari malformation:

- If you are with the patient after surgery, watch for signs of coughing or choking, which may indicate aspiration.
- Observe the patient's breathing, especially how strong the breaths are. If you think there's a problem that suggests apnea, call the nurse.
- The patient should be conscious and able to move both arms and legs. If you notice weakness, call the nurse.

For surgery for syringomyelia:

- Tell the anesthesiologist all the symptoms you've been having, and especially all the medications you've been taking to relieve them—particularly for pain.

For neuroradiological procedures:

- Ask: Who will manage my anesthesia? Will an anesthesiologist be available throughout the procedure?
- Don't bring any metallic objects or credit cards (the magnetic fields will wipe them out) into the MRI room.
- Since it's important that you remain alert enough to respond to any developing symptoms of ischemia, you may have to experience some discomfort during neuroradiological treatment of an AVM and some aneurysms.

CHAPTER 9

• • •

Surgery on Your Heart
and Blood Vessels

• • •

"I did not understand why all these people around my bed were hurting me," wrote *New York Times* columnist A. M. Rosenthal, describing his feelings upon awakening after cardiac bypass surgery. "I was not just frightened but in total, enveloping terror. I felt it not as emotion but as overriding, bottomless pain." Rosenthal's physicians had told him he might be "disoriented by the heavy doses of anesthetics and drugs," but he was evidently not prepared for the "anguish" he experienced of not knowing why he was "being made to suffer so."

Heart surgery, however, does not inevitably cause such a degree of anguish and suffering. Numerous options for postoperative pain control are available that don't have this type of adverse effect, such as patient-controlled analgesia or epidural narcotics (see chapter 2). Unfortunately, even major hospitals may not have the twenty-four-hour pain service necessary for administering and supervising these newer pain-relief techniques. But where such techniques are available, anesthesiology today can provide a much more comfortable experience of open-heart surgery—if you know enough to ask in advance for them.

Much of the surgery performed on the heart and blood vessels is concerned with repairing the effects of arteriosclerosis, a condition in which artery walls become hardened and lined with fatty deposits called plaque. The arteries are narrowed, which means less oxygen-carrying blood can flow through them, and as a result the organs supplied by these vessels—such as the heart, brain, or kidneys—suffer damage due to lack of oxygen.

A major issue for many people with heart or vascular disease is the pain and discomfort they endure in their daily lives. Most cardiac surgery is done to relieve this pain. People with coronary artery disease, for example, have angina—chest pain that occurs in brief spasms, often accompanied by a feeling of suffocation and a terrible sense that death is imminent. Sometimes the heart is so diseased that it can't pump blood out of the lungs, resulting in extreme shortness of breath. People with heart disease sometimes also develop an abnormal heartbeat. We can relieve most of these symptoms with open-heart surgery.

Cardiac and vascular surgery is now a separate field of specialization for anesthesiologists, and many new techniques have been developed in recent years. New diagnostic tests allow us to assess the exact amount of disease present in the heart. Special monitoring techniques make it possible to detect and prevent complications. New drugs enable us to protect the heart and brain from damage during surgery should complications occur. The result has been an improvement in our patients' quality of life, and in some cases an actual extension of their life.

A. M. Rosenthal's terrible experience was probably the result of not being prepared. The most effective way to avoid suffering such as his is to know in advance what questions to ask, what to expect after open-heart surgery, what are the different pain-control methods and their side effects—and what to do if the most effective of these methods are not available.

The first part of this chapter discusses coronary bypass surgery, valve surgery, and heart transplants—all forms of open-heart surgery—and insertion of pacemakers. The second part covers three forms of vascular surgery: carotid endarterectomy, repair of chest and abdominal aortic aneurysms, and bypass surgery for obstructed iliac arteries.

Heart Surgery: Open-Heart Procedures

The coronary arteries supply blood to the heart. When arteriosclerosis develops in these vessels, not enough oxygen reaches the heart muscle due to the diminished blood supply, and you are likely to have angina, feel fluttery in your chest, and experience difficulty breathing when engaging in physical activity. To relieve these symptoms, we perform a surgical procedure in which we graft in a section of a vein or artery, taken from elsewhere in the body, to bypass the occluded, or blocked, vessel, thus increasing the flow of blood to your heart. We also implant arteries taken from inside the chest wall into your heart muscle to improve its blood supply.

When your arteries are clogged and hardened, so too may be the valves of your heart, which means that the flow of blood into and out of the heart is impaired. This clogging and hardening of the heart valves also occurs in people who have had rheumatic fever. We perform valve surgery to replace these diseased valves.

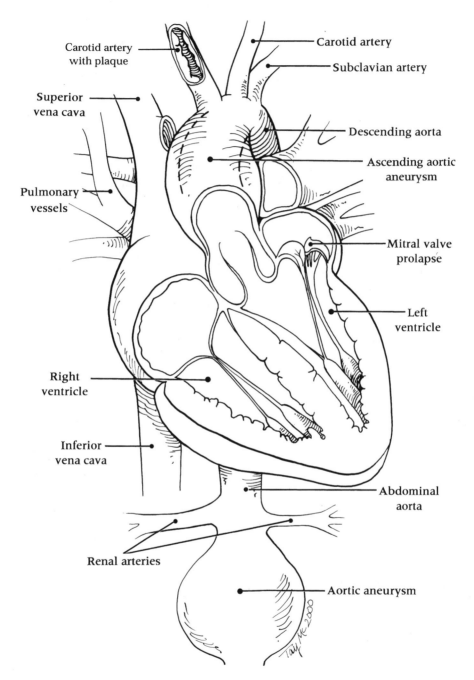

Fig. 12. Heart and major blood vessels, showing aneurysms, mitral valve prolapse, and carotid artery plaque.

Heart transplants are usually required because of a viral infection of the heart or a persistent decrease in flow that cannot be reversed by a bypass alone. Alcoholism, which causes degeneration of the heart muscle, may also make a transplant necessary.

These three heart conditions involve a number of unique considerations for anesthesia, which should be explored during your preoperative consultation with your anesthesiologist.

Preoperative Consultation

During this visit, your anesthesiologist will evaluate your medical condition as a whole. This includes not only the specific nature of your heart ailment but other, related conditions, such as high blood pressure. Patients with heart disease may also have diabetes mellitus, be heavy smokers, and eat high-fat diets that cause disease in other organs. Many are overweight and have stressful life-styles.

Your doctor needs information about all these factors, since they affect the administration of anesthesia—both for special procedures you may require before surgery and during surgery itself. In addition, any of these associated conditions will need to be considered when making plans for pain relief after surgery.

- You should tell your doctor if you:
  —have high blood pressure
  —have diabetes
  —smoke
  —eat a high-fat diet
  —lead a stressful life
  —are asthmatic
  —have a cold
  —have a pacemaker

The medications you're taking will interact with the anesthetics you are given, changing the way the drugs affect your vital processes. In particular, six types of drugs that heart patients often take have significant interactions with anesthetics.

- Tell your doctor if you're taking any of these drugs:
  —Beta blockers (such as atenolol or propranolol). Most patients are taking these drugs to slow a too rapid heartbeat and decrease the heart's need for oxygen. Certain anesthetics given during surgery may amplify this depressant effect,

causing a reduction in blood pressure and decrease in heart rate.

—Antihypertensives (such as clonidine) to treat high blood pressure. Since some antihypertensives have anesthetic effects, the anesthesiologist will need to use less anesthesia to avoid too great a decrease in blood pressure during surgery.

—Calcium channel blockers (such as nifedipine) are also given to depress the heartbeat. Some anesthetics have the same effect, and in combination with a calcium channel blocker can severely reduce the rate and output of the heart.

—Other antiarrhythmics (such as procainamide) can interact with some anesthetics to cause dysrhythmias.

—Diuretics (such as hydrochlorothiazide) can cause low potassium and produce dysrhythmias.

—Vasodilators (such as nitroglycerin), which reduce pressure by dilating the blood vessels, interact with certain anesthetics to cause severe reductions in blood pressure.

—Blood thinners, including aspirin and Coumadin (warfarin), prevent your blood from clotting and should be discontinued prior to surgery.

Finally, during this consultation you should discuss your options for pain control during recovery with your anesthesiologist (see "Recovery from Open-Heart Surgery" below).

Anesthetic-Related Issues for Open-Heart Surgery

Several conditions that are very common in people with heart disease require particularly careful consideration by the anesthesiologist. These include: hypertension (high blood pressure), congestive heart failure, abnormal heartbeats, smoking, diabetes mellitus, and stress resulting from the anticipation of surgery itself.

Hypertension, Congestive Heart Failure, Abnormal Heartbeats. If you have high blood pressure, your anesthesiologist must review and, if necessary, adjust your medications in order to bring your blood pressure to the best state possible prior to surgery. A patient whose blood pressure is not controlled will be at increased risk for other cardiac complications. In addition, if blood pressure rises high enough, vessels in the brain may be affected, causing stroke.

If you have a history of congestive heart failure, the anesthesiologist will need to know specific details of your condition. These should include the last time you were hospitalized (if ever) and your present level of exercise tolerance.

Abnormal heartbeats will result in decreased pumping of blood from the heart during surgery, or even lead to cardiac standstill, in which the heart muscle ceases to contract.

- Tell your anesthesiologist if you notice a fluttering in your chest before surgery or if you have been treated for a fast, irregular heartbeat.

He or she needs to determine the nature of this symptom and try to control it before you have surgery. To make this diagnosis we often give people a Holter monitor to wear. This device provides continuous recording of your heartbeat for twenty-four hours.

Smoking. People with coronary artery disease are often heavy smokers. As I noted in chapter 5, smoking affects the heart as well as the lungs. Since tobacco smoke is a vasoconstrictor (causes the blood vessels to narrow), the heart must work harder to pump blood through the vessels, and because it's diseased it often cannot do so. As a result the heart, kidneys, and brain are damaged because they don't get enough blood. If the coronary arteries are constricted and the heart can't pump strongly enough, the heart muscle itself will die.

Another effect of smoking is that the oxygen in your blood is replaced by carbon monoxide. This increased concentration of carbon monoxide, which further interferes with the delivery of oxygen to your tissues, persists in the blood for a long time.

For these reasons, a two-week smoke-free period before surgery is particularly important for heart patients. If you smoke right up until your operation, the effects of surgery will combine with those of tobacco to cause problems with your breathing and oxygenation. As a result, you may have to stay on a breathing machine (ventilator) for a considerable period.

Unfortunately, I've found that even though most people are intensely afraid of being on these machines, only about half of patients stop smoking even for this brief period. "I'll try," they say, "but you know, it's really difficult." It may be difficult, but not doing it will cause serious problems during and after surgery. And patients who do stop smoking have a much better outcome. They need fewer drugs during surgery and less intensive care afterward.

Diabetes Mellitus. If you have diabetes mellitus, it's extremely important to bring your blood sugar under control before surgery. Most diabetics can do this. If blood sugar is too high during the procedure, you may develop acidosis (excess accumulation of acid in the body). Blood sugar that is too low, on the other hand, can also present problems, since the traditional signs of low blood sugar (hypoglycemia) are difficult to diagnose under anesthesia.

Both the anesthesia and stress from surgery increase blood sugar. Be aware that your blood sugar will vary greatly before, during, and after surgery, and you'll need to carefully monitor your urine sugar or blood sugar and adjust your medication accordingly. Many people taking oral medications find they need to switch to insulin.

- Before surgery, tell your anesthesiologist how well you've been able to control your blood sugar and what adjustments you've had to make in your medications.

Usually, people's anxiety starts to increase about twenty-four hours before surgery, and they need to take more insulin. Since anesthetics administered during surgery affect the body's release of insulin, the drugs you've been taking must be further adjusted after you enter the hospital. We monitor your blood sugar every four to six hours and adjust your insulin accordingly.

Another concern is that heart patients with diabetes often have disease in other blood vessels, possibly including arteriosclerosis of the carotid arteries in the neck, which bring blood to the head. In such a case, these vessels are narrowed and may provide insufficient blood supply to the brain, possibly causing stroke during surgery. Stroke is worse when blood sugar is high.

- Tell your anesthesiologist if you have disease in other blood vessels, especially narrowing of the carotid arteries.

Stress. When Prince Rainier of Monaco needed bypass surgery in December 1994, he became so afraid he might die that he abdicated his throne before entering the hospital. The prospect of having open-heart surgery certainly is frightening, and being scared is stressful. So is surgery itself. Indeed, stress is one of the biggest components of disease. Stress increases risk since it raises blood pressure and heart rate; thus the anesthesiologist's job is to decrease the added stress caused by fear and anxiety—both before and after the procedure. The consequences of not doing so are demonstrated by A. M. Rosenthal's experience.

In fact, our major role is to communicate effectively to relieve people's anxiety when they face heart surgery. The anesthesiologist should see you either in the preadmission testing center weeks before your surgery, on the night before, or on the day of surgery. We talk about the safety of the procedure and the comfort we'll try to provide during it, and we assure you that we'll do everything possible to make you wake up healthier than when you went to sleep.

Sometimes we aren't able to reassure a patient as thoroughly as we'd like with talk, especially since people who have coronary surgery tend to be type A personalities who were very anxious to begin with. In such a case we also give an antianxiety drug, such as a benzodiazepine (Valium) or the shorter-acting midazolam. To that we may add a narcotic to promote a sense of well-being, administered about two hours before surgery. Probably the most effective narcotic for this purpose is morphine, which enhances the effect of the Valium.

Some people don't experience the physiological changes—rapid heartbeat and increased blood pressure—related to stress. But many do, and this can be dangerous.

- It's critically important to tell the anesthesiologist if you're feeling stressed and anxious on the morning of surgery or the night before, so that you can be given a sedative.

When a patient is well sedated, there's much less risk that she or he will develop a heart attack during surgery. Many times I've seen a patient come to the operating room feeling terribly anxious and start to complain of chest pain. At this point we can administer a sedative drug and/or a coronary artery dilator (vasodilator) to relieve the anxiety and the chest pain, before a heart attack occurs.

If necessary, therefore, you should receive a large preoperative dose of sedatives and/or narcotics. As I explained in the introduction (and see chapter 16 for additional discussion), the acute use of narcotics has not proved to be habit-forming. Very few—if any—patients who receive narcotics before surgery become dependent on them.

Special Considerations for Valve Surgery

If you're having valve surgery, additional issues come into play.

- Tell the anesthesiologist if you have had fainting episodes (syncope). If you have this history, special precautions will be needed to prevent decreased blood flow to the brain during surgery.
- Tell the anesthesiologist if you have a history of heart failure. Heart failure must be controlled, if possible, prior to anesthesia and surgery.

- Tell the anesthesiologist if you have experienced an abnormally fast or slow heartbeat.

In patients with valvular disease, a fast heartbeat (which can also be caused by stress) prevents sufficient blood from going to the brain and kidneys because there is not enough time between beats for the blood to fill the ventricle (one of the two larger cavities of the heart that pump blood to the body). Generally, patients with valvular disease need to bring their heartbeat to a normal rate before, during, and after surgery. This is difficult to do before surgery because of the disease in the heart. As a result, we often have to keep the patient in the hospital an extra day or two, postponing surgery until we can bring the heart rate under control.

Special Procedures before Surgery

Patients frequently need one or more diagnostic or therapeutic procedures before open-heart surgery.

Angiogram. Most open-heart-surgery patients need an angiogram, a diagnostic procedure that reveals the degree of disease or narrowing of the heart vessels. The procedure involves threading a catheter through all four chambers of the heart to measure their function and pressures. It is a stressful procedure, and you may need conscious sedation (see the section on conscious sedation in chapter 2).

- Ask whether someone will be available to provide conscious sedation.

Don't hesitate to ask for sedation: remember, there is no reason you should try to bite the bullet. However, it's important to ask in advance, since the person who performs the angiogram cannot also provide sedation. Someone else should be present to administer sedation and monitor its effects.

Angioplasty. In some cases where patients have narrowing of the arteries but do not require surgery, the cardiologist may try instead to dilate the narrowed vessel in a procedure known as angioplasty. A catheter is threaded into the diseased vessel, and a balloon at its end is inflated in order to flatten plaque against the artery wall. Again, this is a stressful procedure requiring conscious sedation.

Depending on the severity of the disease in the heart vessels, complications may occur during angioplasty that will necessitate immediate open-heart surgery. It is, therefore, essential that you have previously provided a detailed history that was placed in your medical record. In such a case, the anesthesiologist who is brought in hurriedly for open-heart surgery will be better able to assess your condition and administer the appropriate anesthetics.

- Ask your cardiologist/internist whether your history is available on your medical record.

Pacemaker Insertion. Sometimes a heart patient develops a complete heart block before open-heart surgery. The normal heart rate of 80 decreases to between 30 and 40, and the patient experiences intermittent fainting episodes because the heart beats abnormally or too slowly to supply enough blood to the brain.

- Tell the anesthesiologist if you have had fainting episodes.

If you have, a temporary pacemaker may have to be inserted or at least be available before surgery begins so that the heart rate can be increased, if necessary, during induction of anesthesia or before the operation is completed. The pacemaker is inserted through a vein under conscious sedation. During this procedure you can feel any change that occurs in your heart rate, and you may become dizzy.

If this happens, tell the person who's monitoring you how you feel. We can give you drugs either to speed or to slow an abnormal heart rate. Alternatively, we can use an electrical defibrillator to convert rhythms that become life-threatening back to normal.

Taking Drugs on the Day of Your Surgery

On the day of your surgery, you should continue with any drugs that the anesthesiologist feels are appropriate, including those for your heart condition. He or she will have determined which specific drugs you need to continue during your preoperative visit. Take them orally with small sips of water right before you go to the operating room, in addition to the sedative or analgesic that will be prescribed by the anesthesiologist to set the stage for smooth induction of the anesthetic.

The Anesthesiologist's Role during Surgery

Different surgical procedures require different types of anesthetics. As we saw in chapter 3, the anesthesiologist plays an extremely complex role during surgery. We administer a combination of drugs, whose doses are carefully calculated to produce the desired effect, and we must recalculate these doses "on the fly" as surgery proceeds, while watching the monitors that tell us what's happening inside your brain and blood vessels.

Bypass Surgery. For bypass surgery we select primarily anesthetics that maintain your heart rate and blood pressure near normal and dilate blood vessels in other areas of the body. One medication can sometimes do all that, but during the procedure we need to have on hand a combination of drugs with different effects.

During bypass surgery we use a cardiopulmonary bypass machine, which circulates the blood outside the body through a pump oxygenator. Usually, the anesthesiologist medically directs the person running the pump while administering drugs, fluids, and blood through it. We also keep track of the perfusion pressure in the pump, which is what keeps the brain functioning.

Valve Surgery. The choice of anesthetics for valve surgery depends on the type of valvular disease the patient has. When the aortic valve (through which the blood flows from the left ventricle into the aorta, the great arterial trunk that carries blood from the heart) is being replaced, the patient may have tachycardia (excessively rapid heart rate), and we need an anesthetic that slows the heart rate. And since the coronary arteries are near the aorta, any increase in heart rate will diminish the blood supply to the heart. In this situation we need an anesthetic that also depresses the heart, decreasing its need for oxygen. For these reasons we use an anesthetic that depresses the heart muscle without causing an increase in the heart rate and also doesn't dilate the chambers of the heart.

Disease of the mitral valve (between the two left-hand chambers of the heart) is of two kinds. In mitral stenosis (narrowing of the valve opening), there also may be tachycardia, so we use an anesthetic that prevents increases in the heart rate. However, with mitral regurgitation (insufficiency of the valve, causing a backflow of blood from the ventricle into the atrium, one of the two smaller cavities), we need an anesthetic that dilates the heart muscle, causing more blood to flow through the valve. But since this type of anesthetic causes tachycardia, we may also need to give a drug that slows the heart, such as a beta blocker.

Valve surgery entails a risk of stroke. To decrease this possibility, we use drugs that protect the brain by suppressing its need for oxygen. Another concern is that patients having valves replaced are at risk of developing neurological problems other than stroke after surgery. Air may get into the heart during the procedure, and after the heart is closed up, the air can travel to the brain. This may cause temporary memory loss after surgery, but the air will disappear as time passes. Tiny pieces of debris from the calcified valves being replaced can also travel through the bloodstream to the brain, also possibly causing memory problems. Rarely, this debris can also result in muscular weakness on either side of the body.

It's the anesthesiologist's and surgeon's job to minimize the amount of possible injury to the brain after valve surgery. This requires paying close attention to emptying air from the blood lines (the tubes that carry blood used in bypass) and careful handling of the heart and its vessels to prevent dislodgement of debris that might travel to the brain. Your surgeon and anesthesiologist will do everything possible to prevent these complications. Some anesthesiologists are now using monitors such as EEG, evoked potential, and Doppler flow probes to see whether these monitors will decrease such complications even more (see chapter 3 for descriptions). If someone asks for your consent to use such monitors in order to help prevent these complications entirely in the future, please consider doing so.

An additional problem in valve surgery is that it is difficult to use monitors inside the heart. We can, however, use a noninvasive monitor, the transesophageal echocardiogram (TEE), which employs sound waves to provide a moving image of your heart during surgery.

Transplants. Viral infection of the heart causes severe problems in maintaining blood pressure and heart rate. For this reason, drops in blood pressure in response to anesthetics are much greater during transplants than in other types of heart surgery, and the anesthesiologist must be prepared to use anesthetics that don't lower blood pressure. She or he must also have ready drugs that raise the pressure, as well as temporary pacemakers to restart the heart if it stops.

- If possible, choose a surgeon and anesthesiologist who perform at least fifty transplants a year. This will ensure that your physicians are prepared to respond to any complications that arise.

As in valve surgery, during heart transplants a noninvasive monitor, such as the TEE, must be used. For this reason, heart transplant patients are more difficult to care for. Since we may not have moment-to-moment feedback from inside the heart, it's important that the transplant be done rapidly. Once the transplant is complete, additional monitors can be placed inside the new heart, to give the anesthesiologist better control over the patient's vital functions during reversal of anesthesia and in the postoperative period.

Recovery from Open-Heart Surgery

The critical need during recovery is to get the heart beating again and restore circulation. The anesthesiologist must reestablish these functions before letting the patient breathe on his or her own. Our goal is to take the breathing tube out of your trachea as soon as possible. The earlier we can do so, the more rapid and complete recovery will be. To determine when extubation can be done, we watch how consistently your blood pressure stays up, how normal your heart rate is, and how well your tissues are being oxygenated.

We also try to get you walking as soon as possible. This means administering pain relief, since when you're in pain you can't sit up or walk. Immobility puts you at risk for deep vein thrombosis, the development of a blood clot in a vein in your leg. The danger is that once this clot has formed during a period of immobility, after you do begin to walk the clot will travel to the lung and obstruct the circulation there. (This happened to former vice president Dan Quayle in 1994 after sitting for twelve hours on a plane.) Effective postoperative pain control is also essential because pain prevents you from breathing deeply, and restricted breathing puts you at risk for pneumonia.

Finally, postoperative pain adds to the stress of heart surgery. Keep in mind that after surgery you can be pain-free, or at the least your pain will be substantially decreased. Knowing the pain-relieving techniques and drugs that are available after open-heart surgery will reduce your anxiety about pain, and you'll experience less stress.

The two most effective ways to control postsurgical pain are patient-controlled analgesia (PCA), in which you administer painkillers to yourself according to your own perception of need, and epidural analgesia, administered through a catheter placed outside the spinal canal (see chapter 2 for complete description).

My own favored form of pain relief to enable patients to walk and breathe deeply soon after surgery is epidural analgesia. This form of pain control also dilates the blood vessels, preventing formation of blood clots in the legs and permitting better wound healing, so the recovery phase is shorter. A rare complication of epidural analgesia is epidural hematoma, or formation of a mass of blood at the site where the needle or catheter is placed. This may happen if the needle or catheter causes bleeding, since the blood is thinned by heparin after surgery and doesn't clot easily. Despite this possibility, I feel that epidural analgesia is the best form of postsurgical pain control. It is particularly effective for pain caused by groin incisions made to remove veins used for bypass surgery.

Some patients aren't comfortable with having needles placed into the spine. For them we use PCA. In any event, patients who receive epidural or patient-controlled analgesia are discharged from the hospital earlier than those given intramuscular narcotics (which are injected into a muscle).

- Before surgery, discuss with your anesthesiologist which method of pain control is best for you. Ask: What postoperative pain control techniques are available? Does the hospital have pumps for patient-controlled analgesia? Is epidural analgesia available? Are physicians educated in pain management available?

If PCA or epidural analgesia is not available, you can still minimize discomfort by staying on top of your pain, through what is known as preemptive analgesia. Once pain starts and becomes severe, it is very difficult to control. Therefore you must make sure you get your medication every four hours, whether you feel you need it or not. Typically, intramuscular analgesia is ordered in your chart every four hours "as needed by patient," so if you don't ask for it, you won't get it.

In addition to being responsible for pain control, the anesthesiologist is often the medical director of respiratory therapy. The respiratory therapist uses techniques ordered by the anesthesiologist to encourage deep breathing and coughing, in order to clear from the lungs mucous secretions that would otherwise remain as a culture medium for bacteria. The therapist may tap on your chest with a hand to stimulate coughing, which helps get rid of retained secretions. Another technique is incentive spirometry. We give you a small device that you blow into against resistance. This opens up areas in the lungs that might be collapsed and encourages deep breathing.

Fast-track open-heart surgery, which speeds up the entire process, is gaining in popularity. Recovery time from anesthesia is decreasing, time in the intensive care unit is kept to a minimum—if patients are sent there at all—and hospital stays are shorter. These changes are another effect of cost-cutting measures taken by hospitals in response to the fixed fees paid by HMOs (see chapter 4).

In general, I believe that the benefits of fast-track surgery outweigh the discomforts. Since your stay in the ICU and later hospital recovery time is shorter, you can return home sooner and recover faster with fewer complications, even though you may experience more discomfort at home initially.

Another Complication of Open-Heart Surgery: Blood Clots

- During the recovery period, pay attention to how long catheters that were inserted for special monitoring are left in your heart.

Usually, catheters are not needed for more than two to three days. If a catheter remains in place for too long, a blood clot will form around it. The danger is that the clot will travel to the brain and cause stroke, or out into the blood vessels and cause a heart attack by occluding a vessel.

- After two to three days, ask that catheters inserted in your heart be removed or replaced if possible.

The importance of this caution is illustrated by the experience of my friend Marty, who entered the hospital for a coronary artery bypass graft procedure. After a successful operation, she was transferred to a surgical ICU, where she became septic (developed a blood infection). This condition required placement of a pulmonary artery catheter, which would enable her doctors to prevent septic shock (circulatory failure caused by severe infection) by monitoring her blood volume and cardiac output.

This particular ICU, however, did not have full-time intensive care doctors. Since the surgeons and anesthesiologists made rounds only when they were not in the operating room, Marty was rarely seen. In fact, her doctors spent so little time with her that they never noticed that her catheter remained in place for six days. Meanwhile, even though she was being treated for sepsis, her temperature remained high, indicating that there was some other, undiscovered source of infection, from which bacteria were entering her blood. This source, it turned out, was a blood clot that had developed in her heart around the catheter.

In the end, Marty had to go back to the OR for a very risky open-heart procedure to have the clot removed. Luckily, she survived without permanent injury except for a chest scar—and some mental scars, as well.

Not only does Marty's story underline the need to ensure that catheters in your heart are removed by the third day; it also highlights the importance of asking whether the hospital has full-time critical care doctors available if you will need intensive care.

Heart Surgery: Permanent Pacemaker Insertion

People who develop abnormal heartbeats, especially heart blocks, and the resulting fainting episodes may require insertion of a permanent pacemaker to increase the heart rate. The pacemaker is placed directly on the outside of the heart, through a hole made in the chest.

During this procedure, several complications may occur. Different heart rhythms or changes in blood pressure may develop, requiring treatment. Electrical equipment in the operating room may interfere with the pacemaker. During placement of the pacemaker, a pneumothorax (accumulation of air in the chest that compresses the lungs, preventing them from expanding) may necessitate insertion of a chest tube to allow the air to exit.

Since these complications require the presence of someone with the skills to treat them, to monitor the electrical devices and insure that they function properly, and to administer conscious sedation during placement of the chest tube, this procedure should never be done without an anesthesiologist present.

Surgery on Blood Vessels

People with arteriosclerosis have disease in other arteries in addition to the coronary arteries. They often need surgery on the carotid and iliac arteries or the aorta.

Carotid Endarterectomy

The carotid arteries supply blood to the brain. Carotid artery disease is usually diagnosed after a person experiences what is known as a transient ischemic attack, resulting from too little oxygen reaching the brain. Such an attack involves temporary weakness in the arm and/or leg on one side of the body, blindness, or slurring of speech. Without treatment, the next stage of carotid artery disease is full-fledged stroke.

- If you experience the symptoms of a transient ischemic attack, consult a physician.

This doctor will perform or request tests to confirm the diagnosis. These tests include a series of angiograms, performed like coronary angiograms under conscious sedation, which identify the extent of the disease and whether surgery will be helpful. Surgery for carotid artery disease involves opening up the artery and removing the fatty plaque from the vessel walls.

Preoperative Consultation

People with carotid artery disease generally also have disease in organs such as the heart and kidneys. These individuals also often lead stressful lives and are heavy smokers who have chronic lung disease.

- Tell the anesthesiologist your complete medical history, particularly the extent of your heart disease.

The anesthesiologist needs all this information because a small number of people having carotid endarterectomies are at an increased risk of developing heart attacks. The anesthesiologist must be prepared to prevent a heart attack from occurring during surgery.

- Tell the anesthesiologist what medications you are taking. This will enable him or her to plan anesthesia management during surgery to maintain your blood pressure.

Awake or Asleep? If you're having a carotid endarterectomy, you'll have to decide whether you want to be awake or asleep during the procedure—that is, have a regional or a general anesthetic.

Some patients prefer to avoid the anxiety of being awake and knowing what's going on. They tell me, "I don't want to know anything about it, I want to be asleep." Others choose to stay awake. These people say, "I want to know if I'm going to be OK."

- Discuss with your anesthesiologist the question of regional versus general anesthetic, so you can decide which will be best for you and cause you the least amount of stress. If you feel being awake will make you crazed, it's probably better to be asleep.

Although there's no difference in ultimate outcome between these two options, patients who choose to remain awake do recover more rapidly, and we have fewer problems controlling their blood pressure. As a result, they may go home sooner.

Use of Drugs on the Day of Surgery

On the day of surgery, you should continue with whatever drugs you've been instructed to take during your preoperative visit.

- Tell the anesthesiologist if you take nitroglycerin for chest pain and have increased the dosage. This information is especially important, since a higher level of nitroglycerin may lower your blood pressure during surgery.

Anesthesia during Surgery

In people with carotid artery disease, any decrease in blood pressure during surgery could cause stroke. Thus the anesthesiologist's most important task during carotid endarterectomy is maintaining the blood flow to the brain. To do this we choose anesthetics that maintain blood pressure. We also often use vasopressors, such as phenylephrine, which stimulate contraction of the capillaries and arteries, to raise the pressure.

In performing the procedure, the surgeon cross-clamps (occludes) the carotid artery before opening it. At this point the anesthesiologist has to interpret the patient's brain function. If you've chosen to remain awake, the anesthesiologist doesn't need a monitor for this, since you can indicate that the brain isn't getting enough blood by saying, "I can't move my arm," for example, or "I can't see." If you've chosen to be asleep, however, the anesthesiologist must rely on ensuring that your blood pressure remains adequate (although a few institutions use EEG or evoked response to monitor the brain). This in itself is a good reason to remain awake during the procedure.

If abnormal brain function occurs, the anesthesiologist advises the surgeon of this so the surgeon can insert a shunt to allow blood flow to continue to the brain during the repair. The surgeon may choose not to place a shunt, in which case the anesthesiologist needs to provide drugs to protect the brain while the artery is occluded.

Recovery

Since myocardial infarction can occur, although rarely, after these procedures, during recovery the anesthesiologist must monitor the heart using an electrocardiogram. When properly placed, this device observes externally the area of the heart that is most vulnerable to developing ischemia (decreased blood supply) or infarct (tissue death due to decreased blood supply resulting from circulatory obstruction).

Patients who have had general anesthesia tend to develop high blood pressure and tachycardia, which puts them at greater risk of myocardial infarction. To prevent this we must administer vasodilators.

Chest and Abdominal Aortic Aneurysms

Like the coronary and carotid arteries, the aorta can become diseased with arteriosclerosis. This weakens the arterial wall and causes the vessel to dilate abnormally, creating a pouch called an aneurysm. If the dilation is large enough, the vessel will rupture, causing rapid death. Surgery is necessary to prevent rupture.

Depending on the aneurysm's size and location, the complications of the procedure and its outcomes vary. The closer the aneurysm is to the heart, the greater the risk, since the blood flow to the heart will be impaired while the surgery proceeds.

Ascending Aneurysms

Aneurysms that occur above the point on the aorta where the carotid arteries branch off to the head are known as ascending aneurysms. Repairing them requires clamping arteries, to temporarily suspend blood flow to the brain, and use of a cardiopulmonary bypass machine. Although it's optimal to monitor the brain during repair of an ascending aneurysm, only a few medical centers do so. However, the majority of patients recover satisfactorily without this specialized monitoring.

Descending Aneurysms

Descending aneurysms are those that occur below the branching off of the carotid arteries. Since the repair can be done without cardiopulmonary bypass, complications are fewer. We do need to monitor the functions of other organs that can be affected by the clamping of the aorta.

Thus we observe urine output; if the amount decreases, we administer a diuretic such as mannitol or furosemide to stimulate kidney function until the aorta is reopened. On rare occasions, when the clamp must be left on for a long period of time, the blood flow to the spinal cord may be decreased due to increased pressure on the cord exerted by the clamp. In such a case the surgeon may place a cerebrospinal fluid (CSF) drain in the lower spine to decrease pressure on the spinal cord and help prevent paraplegia. Monitors, such as evoked potential, have been used to check the function of the spinal cord, but are of limited value because they may produce false negative results. There is certainly no danger in this type of monitoring, however, and it may be helpful, so it can't hurt to ask whether it can be done.

- Ask: Can my spinal cord function be monitored by evoked potential?

Abdominal Aneurysms

This type of aneurysm occurs further down, between the diaphragm and the point in the pelvis where the aorta branches into the iliac arteries

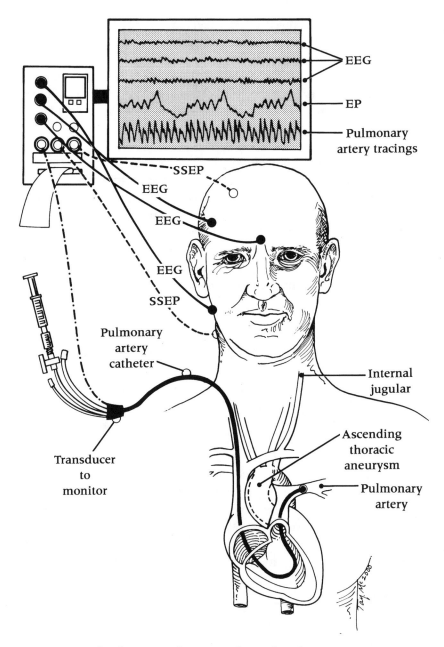

Fig. 13. *Specialized monitors for repair of ascending thoracic aneurysm: electroencephalogram, evoked potentials, and pulmonary artery pressure (Swan-Ganz catheter).*

supplying the legs. Abdominal aneurysms are the least risky to repair. During surgery the anesthesiologist is primarily concerned with spinal cord and kidney function.

Anesthesia during Surgery

For repair of an aneurysm, the anesthesiologist chooses anesthetics that maintain blood flow to your vital organs without decreasing pressure. We also select drugs that protect the heart, brain, and spinal cord.

Special monitors to determine the effectiveness of these anesthetics, including a pulmonary artery catheter, are commonly used because of the great changes in fluid and blood volume and the large fluctuations in pressure that occur. When the surgeon clamps the aorta, the pressure above the clamp becomes extremely high and can damage the heart and brain. Then when the clamp is removed, the pressure becomes low, which can also damage the heart and brain. The monitors help us prevent and treat these high and low pressures.

- Ask: Will the monitor will be placed before or after I'm asleep? Placing this monitor involves inserting a needle into your upper chest and lower neck. If you feel extremely anxious and would prefer not to be awake during this procedure, you can request that it not be done until after anesthesia is induced. If the monitor must be placed while you're still awake, request appropriate sedation until you no longer feel anxious.

Bypass Surgery for Occluded Iliac Arteries

The iliac arteries (which supply the pelvis and legs) can also become blocked due to arteriosclerosis. Most often we do bypass surgery to relieve pain in the legs that occurs on walking, which is caused by a decreased blood supply that can't provide the additional oxygen the muscles require during exercise. We also perform bypass surgery for ulcerations on the legs or gangrene in the toes caused by ischemia, usually secondary to diabetes.

The procedure involves inserting an artificial blood vessel, made of Teflon or another plastic, to channel the blood flow from a point above the occlusion to a point below it.

Preoperative Consultation and Anesthesia-Related Issues

Like those who come for open-heart and carotid procedures, patients who need iliac bypass generally have high blood pressure and angina. They are overweight, live stressful lives, and smoke. Thus the anesthesiologist's concerns during the preliminary consultation, and the anesthesia-related issues to consider, are the same as for these other procedures (see the sections "Anesthetic-Related Issues for Open-Heart Surgery" and, under "Carotid Endarterectomy," "Preoperative Consultation" and "Awake or Asleep?" above).

Special Procedures before Surgery

Some special procedures needed before iliac bypass surgery involve anesthesiology.

Diagnostic Angiography. To determine how much of the iliac artery is occluded, you will need angiography. A catheter is fed into an artery, dye is injected into the catheter, and an x-ray is made. The blocked sections of the artery, into which the dye cannot flow, are highlighted on the film. The procedure is painful, and requires conscious sedation.

Sometimes the patient has an allergic reaction to the dye, or it may cause the blood vessels to go into spasm. These reactions can be treated with appropriate drugs. If you have previously had a reaction to dye, you should tell the anesthesiologist this.

Other Tests. Before iliac bypass surgery we also need to assess the extent of disease in the heart and carotids, to predict the likelihood of complications, such as heart attack or stroke. You may, therefore, have a preoperative echocardiogram (an ultrasound procedure) or stress test. An abnormal echocardiogram signals the anesthesiologist to monitor the heart more closely using specialized monitors during surgery. If, using these monitors, we see the heart function decrease, we can give drugs or fluids to restore it. The results of the stress test tell us how much risk there will be during the procedure.

Anesthesia during Surgery

Since iliac bypass surgery does not involve major arteries near the heart, it does not require a general anesthetic. Not only is a regional anesthetic thought to increase blood flow to the legs, but the epidural catheter can be left in place after surgery so that pain-relieving drugs can be administered through it. This allows you to get up and walk sooner. Early ambulation in turn promotes better wound healing and diminishes the risk of deep vein thrombosis.

During surgery the anesthesiologist is concerned with preventing heart attack and stroke. If you're awake, you're likely to be scared, which increases stress and consequently the heart rate. Regional anesthetics can also interfere with the blood supply to the heart and brain because they decrease blood pressure.

We use special monitors to detect decreased blood flow to the heart. If the patient is awake, we don't need to monitor the brain since we can ask you questions about how you feel (see the section "Anesthesia during Surgery" under "Carotid Endarterectomy," above). However, a significant number of patients refuse a regional for this procedure and request a general anesthetic. For them, we need to use a brain monitor.

- I know it's frightening to be awake, but be aware that you can also receive sedation to help you stay calm. Remember that regional anesthesia has advantages over general anesthesia.

Recovery

Your choices for pain control during recovery depend on which anesthetic technique you had for surgery. If you had a regional, you can continue to receive narcotics through the epidural catheter, by either self-administered or physician-administered injection. If you had general anesthesia, however, your choices are limited to patient-controlled analgesia or oral narcotics (for details see chapter 2).

Because people who require iliac bypass also have disease in other body systems, we monitor them carefully in the recovery room. Most heart attacks associated with this procedure occur after the operation, as a result of pain and the stress of undergoing surgery, which leads to high blood pressure and an increase in the heart rate. So the anesthesiologist must control stress using sedation and analgesia, as well as the equally important technique of reassurance.

Optimally, you should be monitored for at least twenty-four hours after surgery. If blood pressure or heart rate changes significantly within the initial twenty-four hours, another twenty-four hours of monitoring would be useful to make sure these symptoms don't recur. However, many patients are no longer monitored for this length of time. Fortunately, most recover satisfactorily with shorter monitoring periods.

Complications

The major complications after iliac bypass surgery are myocardial infarction and stroke, due to narrowing of the arteries supplying blood to the heart and brain or to occlusion of the new bypass grafts by clots. These complications can be avoided by meticulous monitoring during and after surgery and in the critical care unit.

Summary: Questions and Points to Remember

- Tell your doctor if you have high blood pressure, diabetes, a cold, or a pacemaker; if you smoke; eat a high-fat diet; lead a stressful life; or are asthmatic.
- Tell your doctor if you're taking beta blockers, antihypertensive drugs, calcium channel blockers, other antiarrhythmics, diuretics, vasodilators, or blood thinners.
- Tell your anesthesiologist if you notice a fluttering in your chest before surgery or if you have been treated for a fast, irregular heartbeat.
- It's critically important to tell the anesthesiologist if you're feeling stressed and anxious on the morning of surgery or the night before, so that you can be given a sedative.
- If you have diabetes mellitus: Tell your anesthesiologist before surgery how well you've been able to control your blood sugar and what adjustments you've had to make in your medications.
- Before heart surgery, tell your anesthesiologist if you have disease in other blood vessels, especially narrowing of the carotid arteries.
- Before valve surgery, tell the anesthesiologist if you have had fainting episodes (syncope).
- Before valve surgery, tell the anesthesiologist if you have a history of heart failure.
- Before valve surgery, tell the anesthesiologist if you have experienced an abnormally fast or slow heartbeat.
- Before an angiogram, ask whether someone will be available to provide conscious sedation.
- Before an angioplasty, ask your cardiologist/internist whether your history is available on your medical record.
- If you're having a pacemaker inserted, tell the anesthesiologist if you have had fainting episodes.
- For a heart transplant: If possible, choose a surgeon and anesthesiologist who perform at least fifty transplants a year.
- Before open-heart surgery, discuss with your anesthesiologist which method of pain control is best for you.
- Ask: What postoperative pain control techniques are available? Does the hospital have pumps for patient-controlled analgesia? Is epidural analgesia available? Are physicians educated in pain management available?

- During recovery from open-heart surgery, pay attention to how long catheters that were inserted for special monitoring are left in your heart.
- After two to three days, ask that catheters inserted in your heart be removed or replaced if possible.
- If you experience the symptoms of a transient ischemic attack, consult a physician.
- If you have carotid artery disease, tell the anesthesiologist your complete medical history, particularly the extent of your heart disease. Tell the anesthesiologist what medications you are taking.
- Before a carotid endarterectomy, discuss with your anesthesiologist the question of regional versus general anesthetic, so you can decide which will be best for you and cause you the least amount of stress. If you feel being awake will make you crazed, it's probably better to be asleep.
- Before carotid endarterectomy, tell the anesthesiologist if you take nitroglycerin for chest pain and have increased the dosage.
- If you're having surgery for a descending aneurysm, ask: Can my spinal cord function be monitored by evoked potential?
- Before repair of any type of aneurysm, ask: Will the pulmonary artery catheter be placed before or after I'm asleep?
- If you feel extremely anxious and would prefer not to be awake during placement of this monitor, you can request that it not be done until after anesthesia is induced.
- If the monitor must be placed while you're still awake, request appropriate sedation until you no longer feel anxious. I know it's frightening to be awake during iliac bypass surgery, but be aware that you can also receive sedation to help you stay calm. Remember that regional anesthesia has advantages over general anesthesia.

• • •

CHAPTER 10

Chest Surgery

• • •

During the 1990s, advances in equipment and in anesthetic techniques led to more diagnostic and treatment procedures being performed in the chest cavity. Thoracic surgery (from the term "thorax," or chest) ranges from bronchoscopy and mediastinoscopy, relatively minor diagnostic procedures, to major operations such as removal of a lung.

Because patients who need these chest procedures are older and commonly smokers, anesthesia for them is frequently complicated by preexisting lung disease, such as chronic bronchitis, emphysema, and asthma, that is quite hard to control. (See chapter 5 for details on how tobacco use complicates anesthesia.) These patients require preparation, sometimes weeks in advance, as well as absolute vigilance on the part of the anesthesiologist during the procedure itself.

Bronchoscopy

There are two types of bronchoscopy: flexible bronchoscopy and rigid bronchoscopy. Both involve insertion of tubular instruments into the bronchi, or air passages of the lungs, which branch off the trachea, or windpipe.

A flexible bronchoscope is a fiberoptic tube with a light at the end that is inserted into the mouth and down into the trachea to directly observe the bronchi. We perform flexible bronchoscopy to diagnose a variety of lung conditions, including pneumonia that hasn't cleared up after treatment; a possible tumor, as indicated by abnormal chest x-rays; and infection, suggested by a chronic cough. Flexible bronchoscopy can be quite uncomfortable and often requires deep sedation and a great deal of topical anesthesia.

An initial diagnostic technique is to inject saline solution into the bronchoscope, then aspirate it out. The aspirated fluid brings with it cells from the lungs that are cultured to diagnose tuberculosis or pneumonia.

Sometimes abnormal cells that may be cancerous are obtained. Depending on the results, the surgeon or pulmonologist will then take biopsies of tissue to confirm the diagnosis. These biopsies may cause bleeding or produce tissue injury, such as perforation or obstruction of the airways. The anesthesiologist must be prepared to increase the concentration of oxygen that the patient is inhaling, should complications occur.

The type of anesthesia we use for flexible bronchoscopy will depend on your decision as to whether you want to be awake or asleep. Most physicians prefer that patients be awake so that, when asked to breathe deeply or cough, they can do so. But if you'd rather be asleep, the anesthesiologist can perform these maneuvers.

- If you've agreed to remain conscious during flexible bronchoscopy, and you feel you need more sedation, don't hesitate to ask for it.

We administer anesthesia for flexible bronchoscopy by inhalation of nebulized local anesthetics, by spraying the drug directly into the trachea, or by performing nerve blocks around the trachea. If you've decided to remain conscious, I suggest that you request the inhalation method, for I find that patients tolerate inhalation more easily and can therefore be more cooperative. Best of all is combining inhalation with topical anesthesia, in the form of viscous lidocaine. This technique avoids sudden coughing spasms as the spray of local anesthetic hits the tissues, as well as the experience of having needles in your neck.

- If you're scheduled for a bronchoscopy under conscious sedation and local anesthesia, request an inhalation technique or inhalation combined with topical anesthesia.

Rigid bronchoscopy is used to remove foreign bodies, such as peanuts, from the airways of children and adults. For this procedure, in which the surgeon inserts a rigid tube directly into the trachea, you need general anesthesia.

Both types of bronchoscopy can trigger attacks of asthma or other complications, which often must be treated aggressively right on the spot by the anesthesiologist.

- If you have asthma or another preexisting lung condition—and the situation is not an emergency—you must see your internist and/or anesthesiologist at least a week before surgery so that wheezing and any infection can be brought under control.

Mediastinoscopy

The mediastinum is the area of the chest that contains the tissues and organs lying between the lungs—the heart, major blood vessels, trachea, esophagus, thymus, lymph nodes, and others. Mediastinoscopy uses a specially designed fiberoptic mediastinoscope to diagnose tumors in this area; to look for suspicious lymph nodes that may indicate either lung cancer or lymphoma, a neoplasm of the lymph tissue; and to diagnose thymoma, a tumor of the thymus that is associated with an autoimmune condition called myasthenia gravis.

The mediastinoscope is inserted through an incision in the base of the neck, into the area where the major vessels emerge from and pass into the heart, permitting observation and biopsy of this area. Since mediastinoscopy is an extremely painful procedure, it is almost always performed under general anesthesia unless there is an absolute medical contraindication.

- If your anesthesiologist or surgeon suggests that you have a mediastinoscopy done under conscious sedation and local anesthesia, ask for general anesthesia instead, unless your medical condition contraindicates it.

The anesthetic concerns for mediastinoscopy are the same as for bronchoscopy: preexisting conditions, particularly bronchitis, chronic cough, and asthma, must be controlled as well as possible before the procedure can be performed. A number of complications are possible. One is occlusion (blockage) of the trachea, which the anesthesiologist must recognize and correct immediately; another is bleeding from damage to the major vessels or from a biopsy. A third is compression of a major vessel, which can lead to decreased blood flow to the brain. A fourth is pneumothorax (an accumulation of air in the chest that compresses the lungs and prevents them from expanding), which can result in hypoxia (insufficient oxygen supply to the tissues). The anesthesiologist treats pneumothorax by inserting a tube into the chest through which the air can escape, allowing the lungs to expand. A final possible complication is vocal cord paralysis caused by injury to the nerve that travels through the mediastinum and supplies the cord.

Thoracoscopy

Thoracoscopy is a technique for diagnosing abnormalities in the pleura, the membrane that lines the lungs and the inner wall of the chest cavity.

We perform thoracoscopy when there is infection and accumulations of fluid in the pleura as a result of various diseases, as well as to determine the stage of progression of cancer.

Thoracoscopy can also be a form of treatment for a pneumothorax resulting from what is known as bullous emphysema. In this condition, the walls of the air sacs in the lungs are destroyed, and large balloonlike structures protrude from the lung surface. A laser is inserted inside the tube and used to obliterate the bullae in order to prevent them from rupturing and creating the pneumothorax.

For a thoracoscopy, the fiberoptic tube is inserted through an incision made between two ribs on one side. Since this procedure is not as painful as mediastinoscopy, it's usually done under conscious sedation and local anesthesia, in the form of intercostal nerve blocks (placed between the ribs). These blocks also anesthetize the pleura, which contains many pain fibers. If the patient's preexisting lung disease causes much coughing, we can place a stellate ganglion block to suppress the cough reflex. (The stellate ganglion is a mass of nerve cells located at the side of the neck.)

During this procedure, we insufflate (blow) air into the chest to separate the pleura from the chest wall, allowing access for the surgeon. Doing so, however, creates a partial pneumothorax, which the anesthesiologist observes closely. If this pneumothorax expands too much, the anesthesiologist may be forced to provide general anesthesia in order to control the patient's breathing.

Thoracotomy

The term "thoracotomy" means opening the chest cavity by means of an incision, which is generally done to resect (remove) lung tumors. These tumors may be primary, meaning that they originate in the lung, or metastatic, meaning that the cancer originated at another site. Primary lung tumors, usually the consequence of years of smoking, are generally large at the time they are diagnosed and thus require major lung resections. This may mean lobectomy, resection of a lobe of a lung, or pneumonectomy, resection of the entire lung.

Before surgery can be done, chronic infections, cough, and wheezing must be treated. Another type of preparation consists of measures to prevent postoperative atelectasis (collapse of the lung). A nurse or respiratory therapist usually instructs the patient how to breathe deeply, cough, and practice blowing into a bottle against resistance.

- If you're scheduled for a thoracotomy, ask that a respiratory therapist teach you how to prevent postoperative respiratory complications.

Anesthesia for these patients is complex and demanding, often requiring that we use arterial lines and central venous pressure monitors to monitor blood gases and detect cardiac abnormalities, such as right heart failure. We use a special technique of pushing a regular endotracheal tube down the right bronchus, past where the left one branches off, to enable only the right lung to breathe. The left lung, the one being operated on, remains still, allowing the surgeon to work unhampered. Alternatively, we can use a special endotracheal tube that allows us to occlude the bronchus of either lung.

During one-lung breathing, as this technique is called, the level of oxygen in the patient's blood may drop too low, compelling the anesthesiologist to perform other special maneuvers to prevent hypoxia. For example, we may give continuous positive airway pressure (CPAP) to the lung being operated on, keeping it continuously inflated without causing movement. Still another technique, positive end-expiratory pressure (PEEP), maintains the air pressure at the end of an exhalation instead of letting it return to normal. The pressure holds the tiny air sacs in the lungs open, allowing more oxygen to enter the blood.

Recovery after thoracotomy can be difficult, since so many patients have chronic lung disease. Most develop atelectasis after surgery and need aggressive respiratory therapy: chest percussion by a nurse or respiratory therapist and antibiotics if infection develops. Equally important are the patient's own efforts to breathe, putting the respiratory therapist's lesson into practice by using the blow bottle and other maneuvers. The anesthesiologist's responsibility here is to ensure that the patient can breathe without pain, which is transmitted by the pain fibers in the pleura as the lungs expand on the inhalation.

Many physicians give intercostal nerve blocks to decrease this pain caused by deep breathing, but my preference is thoracic epidural anesthesia, for which we place the catheter between the shoulder blades. Nerve blocks, if misplaced, can create a pneumothorax, which can lead to atelectasis and pneumonia (since infection is likely to develop when the lungs don't function adequately). Moreover, these blocks wear off after six to twenty-four hours and must be repeated, which increases further the chance of pneumothorax. With an epidural catheter in place, narcotics can be supplied continuously for up to three days, avoiding not only

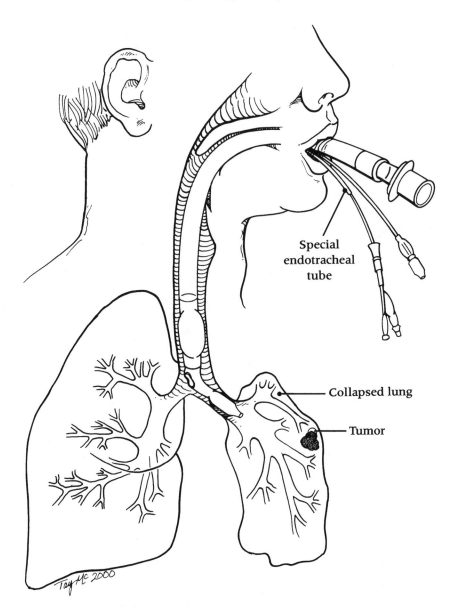

Fig. 14. Lungs, showing one-lung breathing with special endotracheal tube. Left lung is collapsed and right lung is being ventilated.

the risk of pneumothorax but the patient experiencing pain as the block wears off. An intrapleural catheter can also be inserted between the two layers of the pleura and left in place for injection of local anesthetics and/ or narcotics.

- If you've had a thoracotomy and you experience severe pain while breathing, ask for a thoracic epidural anesthetic.

Summary: Questions and Points to Remember

- If you've agreed to remain conscious during flexible bronchoscopy and you feel you need more sedation, don't hesitate to ask for it.
- If you're scheduled for a bronchoscopy under conscious sedation and local anesthesia, request an inhalation technique or inhalation combined with topical anesthesia.
- If you have asthma or another preexisting lung condition—and the situation is not an emergency—you must see your internist and/or anesthesiologist at least a week before surgery so that wheezing and any infection can be brought under control.
- If your anesthesiologist or surgeon suggests that you have a mediastinoscopy done under conscious sedation and local anesthesia, ask for general anesthesia instead, unless your medical condition contraindicates it.
- If you're scheduled for a thoracotomy, ask that a respiratory therapist teach you how to prevent postoperative respiratory complications.
- If you've had a thoracotomy and you experience severe pain while breathing, ask for a thoracic epidural anesthetic.

CHAPTER 11

• • •

Transplants

• • •

In 1995 the actor Larry Hagman, who had starred as J. R. in *Dallas*, was diagnosed with a liver tumor and put on a waiting list for a liver transplant. Three weeks later, he had surgery on the tumor to buy him extra time while he was waiting. During this entire period, he remained in good health and spirits, according to his publicist. Two weeks after the surgery, Hagman received a donated liver, and by 1997 had recovered so well that he was starring in a new TV series.

Hagman's case is an exception. More representative is that of football great Walter Payton, who discovered in 1999 that he had primary sclerosing cholangitis, a rare liver disease, and needed a transplant to survive. Sadly, Payton did not receive a liver in time, and he died later that same year. Had he received one, when the anesthesiologist saw him for the first time in the intensive care unit, he probably would have been near death's door.

Nowadays, organ transplants are considered routine, and more and more people are lining up for these procedures. But their hopes, unfortunately, are often thwarted by the limited availability of donated organs. Indeed in many countries rumors circulate of organs being sold on the black market. This market is fueled by the desperation of patients for whom someone else's liver or kidney represents the last chance for survival.

In the United States, the United Network for Organ Sharing (UNOS), a nonprofit agency, coordinates the distribution of donated organs to recipients. Before 2000, its policy was to offer available organs locally first. If no local matching patient was found, the organ was offered regionally, then nationally. Starting in 2000, organs were offered more broadly across regions. The new policy was designed to even out the waiting times among geographical regions. Conceivably, this change might have made a difference in the fate of Payton, in Illinois, as compared to that of Hagman, in California.

Under this distribution system, patients on the waiting list, surgeons, and anesthesiologists are constantly on the alert for impending transplant operations. This means that patients who are high on the list must have preoperative consultations in advance, so they will be prepared when an organ does become available.

Patients who need organ transplants are by definition in very poor medical condition, and all aspects of their care require close attention. Fortunately, UNOS provides counseling by social workers and/or psychologists to prepare patients and their families for the surgery. Included is information regarding what to expect from the anesthesiologist. In addition, a nurse coordinator follows the patient during the wait for the organ, so she or he has all the information that the anesthesiologist needs.

Partly because they have received information from UNOS, most transplant patients and their families don't ask to see the anesthesiologist preoperatively. In fact, these patients are so desperate that they tend not to ask many questions at all. But the complexity of the procedure and its potential for major complications make a preoperative anesthesia visit by family members mandatory. Families should make sure that the anesthesiologist knows the patient's history, including important aspects of management and drug treatments to date. Beyond this, as I've explained before, even just knowing what to expect can reduce both the patient's and the family's anxiety level considerably.

- During the preoperative consultation, ask: What types of invasive monitors will you use, and will you place them before or after you induce anesthesia?

Often transplant patients are so sick that we must place the monitors before surgery, which means administering sedation and analgesia. But because their condition prevents us from giving large enough doses of the drugs, we may not be able to completely relieve pain and stress. It's better for the patient to know this in advance, so there are no surprises.

- If the patient's condition allows it, request that the monitors be placed after anesthesia is induced.

This chapter describes kidney and liver transplants; for a discussion of heart transplants, see chapter 9.

Kidney Transplants

Kidney transplants are the most frequent type of organ transplantation performed in this country. Patients have end-stage kidney disease and depend on dialysis to live. (Dialysis is a process that separates out of the blood the waste products that the kidneys are unable to excrete.) In most cases the transplant is extremely successful; the new kidney functions well, and the patient no longer requires dialysis.

Kidneys for transplantation come either from a donor who has died (these are called cadaveric transplants) or from a living relative of the patient. Living-related-donor transplants are more successful, since the new kidney is more compatible with the patient's tissues than one from a nonrelative would be.

Children require kidney transplants mostly in cases of infection or congenital abnormality, such as polycystic kidney disease (an inherited disorder that causes a deterioration in kidney function, beginning either in childhood or during adulthood). Without the transplant, the child would not grow normally but would instead become dwarfed. Adults commonly need a new kidney as a result of diabetes mellitus; cancer; the effects of chemotherapy drugs and certain antibiotics; endocrine abnormalities; drug use, particularly heroin; infection; congenital abnormalities, including polycystic disease; and autoimmune diseases, such as lupus. Adults also often need transplants because of arteriosclerosis, which eventually leads to high blood pressure that severely damages the kidneys.

Anesthesia for kidney transplants can be quite difficult, since patients are in such bad shape. However, even for cadaveric transplants, many patients are notified at least forty-eight hours before the actual surgery, which leaves enough time for adequate preparation. With living donors, there is plenty of time.

Preoperative Consultation

Be prepared to give the anesthesiologist a list of all your diseases, as well as the medications you take to control them. Tell him or her when you were last dialyzed, and note any particular problems you've had recently, such as a cough or increased bleeding from minor injuries.

It's also important to describe your previous experience with anesthesia. Patients on dialysis have had surgical procedures called arteriovenous grafts, in which an artery is fed into a vein in the wrist to provide a place to insert the tubes from the dialysis machine. Since these patients have had several such procedures, they know how they react to anesthesia.

- If you have been notified that a kidney is available, ask to see your anesthesiologist as soon as possible.

Patients scheduled for a kidney transplant require dialysis within forty-eight hours of surgery. Before inducing anesthesia, the anesthesiologist must know whether or not the patient's fluid volume (the amount of blood circulating in the body) is adequate and what the electrolyte levels were after dialysis. Electrolytes, substances required for conduction of nerve impulses, must be kept in precise balance. Too high or too low a potassium level, for example, could cause the heart to stop.

Patients with renal disease are usually anemic, so we give them erythropoetin (a hormone that stimulates red cell production in the bone marrow) to boost their blood count before surgery. Often their blood coagulation is impaired, so we must be careful to prevent bleeding when we place invasive monitors. Since their immune systems are impaired as well, we must take great care to provide sterile conditions as we place these monitors and any intravenous lines. Frequently, these patients are also on chronic steroids, which the anesthesiologist will continue to give during the operation; and since steroids suppress the immune system, they increase the need for sterile conditions, so we wear sterile gloves and gowns during invasive procedures.

Anesthesia during Surgery

In many patients with kidney disease, the stomach does not empty normally, so we consider them to have a full stomach. This means managing the airway carefully to prevent aspiration of stomach contents into the lungs. Patients are also hypertensive (have high blood pressure), so we must be prepared to treat wide swings in blood pressure. And throughout the procedure, we closely monitor electrolytes and blood sugar so these too can be controlled.

In some cases there's no time for the erythropoetin to have its maximum effect before a kidney becomes available, so some anesthesiologists may suggest that you have a transfusion right before surgery, in order to assure that adequate oxygen reaches your tissues during anesthesia. However, I believe that in most cases a transfusion is not necessary, since your body has developed compensatory mechanisms to provide adequate oxygenation.

- Tell the anesthesiologist in advance that you prefer not to receive a transfusion before surgery.

In inducing anesthesia, we give a lower dose of anesthetic drugs than usual, since anesthesia may have a greater effect when kidney function is impaired. Since the kidneys are unable to excrete some intravenous drugs, we may need to use inhalation drugs or intravenous drugs that aren't excreted by the kidneys. Yet we must use the inhalation drugs cautiously, since dialysis may have left the patient with low fluid volume, and the drugs increase the risk of low blood pressure.

Because of the patient's potentially impaired blood coagulation, we usually can't give regional anesthesia, such as a lumbar epidural (placed in the low back), for this would create a risk of bleeding around the epidural needle. The result could be formation of a hematoma (mass of blood) that would compress the spinal cord and cause paralysis. Therefore most patients have general anesthesia.

Once the new kidney has been inserted, to ensure plenty of circulation through it we elevate the patient's blood pressure, either with fluids or with a vasopressor drug, such as dopamine, which helps the kidney survive in its new host. We also give diuretic drugs to help promote urine formation and excretion.

Recovery

Postoperatively, kidney transplant patients need adequate pain relief, which is difficult to provide, since the kidneys' ability to excrete narcotics is still impaired, and too large a dose would remain in the patient's body, becoming toxic. So we give lower doses, usually by means of patient-controlled analgesia. Since giving regional anesthesia through an epidural may increase the risk of bleeding around the spine, we give PCA through an intravenous catheter in the back of the hand. If PCA is unavailable, you will have to take oral narcotics, which can also relieve the pain completely.

- Ask: Is PCA available for postoperative pain relief?

Since the patient is now receiving drugs to suppress the immune system so that it will accept the new kidney, sterile conditions must be maintained. This means, among other things, that visitors should wear masks and gowns.

Liver Transplants

By the late 1990s, liver transplants were not only safer than ever before but more accessible (although livers were the scarcest donated organ). People who need new livers have end-stage liver disease resulting from hepatitis B or C, cirrhosis due to alcoholism, drug-induced liver damage, cancer, congenital abnormalities, and various autoimmune disorders.

These patients, like those who need kidney transplants, have medical conditions that must be treated before their surgery. Their damaged livers make them unable to manufacture the proteins necessary to metabolize and excrete drugs. They also have ascites (an abnormal accumulation of protein and electrolyte-rich fluid that seeps from the liver out into the abdominal cavity). This condition drains the body of electrolytes, which must be replaced before the transplantation.

Liver transplant patients have many other problems as well. Circulating toxins that accumulate because the liver is unable to clear them from the blood may result in impaired brain function, which can lead to brain swelling and seizures. In addition, blood coagulation is abnormal; lung abnormalities may result in inadequate oxygen in the blood; malnutrition and fluctuating blood sugar are serious problems; and, since liver disease adversely affects the kidneys, patients may also have impaired renal function.

Preoperative Consultation

Given this panoply of problems, the anesthesiologist needs to assess all your major body systems before surgery. As I explained above, this consultation must occur ahead of time, before a liver becomes available, which means that during the evaluation the anesthesiologist looks for conditions that are likely to worsen while you are waiting. This enables him or her to be prepared for what your condition will be when the liver is obtained.

During the preoperative consultation, the anesthesiologist will assess your neurological function, electrolytes, blood count, and kidney function, and obtain an arterial blood gas measurement to determine how well your blood is oxygenated. She or he will also look for distention of your abdomen due to ascites, to see if this mass of fluid is likely to compress your lungs and further impair oxygenation. Rarely, the anesthesiologist may ask the surgeon to drain some of the ascites right before surgery in order to improve your breathing.

Most people who require a liver transplant are so sick that they are unable to participate in their own care, so they need a family member or friend to act as an advocate.

- If your friend or family member is waiting for a liver transplant, accompany him or her to the preoperative consultation with the anesthesiologist and bring all pertinent medical information.

Anesthesia during Surgery

During liver transplant surgery, the anesthesiologist's most important concern is keeping up with blood loss. We may need to replace as much as four times the patient's blood volume, so multiple large-diameter catheters are routinely inserted to rapidly infuse fluids and blood as necessary. Optimally, we use a cell saver to salvage, clean, and reinfuse your own blood during the procedure, thus avoiding the risks of a transfusion. In cases of infection or malignancy, however, your own blood can't be used, and you will need a transfusion.

The anesthesiologist must constantly monitor the patient to be sure that the anesthetic drugs remain effective, since the large shifts in fluid volume as the operation proceeds might dilute their effects. At the same time, we monitor the patient's electrolytes, hematocrit (the concentration of red blood cells in the blood), blood sugar, and clotting factors (substances manufactured by the liver that are responsible for clotting), so we can replace these as necessary.

Once the new liver is in place and blood begins to circulate through it, the anesthesiologist must be prepared to treat abnormal heart rhythms, low blood pressure, and electrolyte imbalances, all the result of toxins being flushed out of the new liver.

Recovery

After surgery, we continue to replace fluid volume, electrolytes, blood sugar, and clotting factors as necessary. We relieve pain with intravenous narcotics, since regional anesthesia could increase bleeding. Since the patient is now receiving immunosuppressants, we must maintain sterile conditions.

- If the patient seems to be in pain, or you notice that the patient is bleeding, is not breathing properly, has a decreased level of consciousness, or is confused, notify the nurse.

Summary: Questions and Points to Remember

- During the preoperative consultation, ask: What types of invasive monitors will you use, and will you place them before or after you induce anesthesia?
- If the patient's condition allows it, request that the monitors be placed after anesthesia is induced.

For kidney transplants:

- If you have been notified that a kidney is available, ask to see your anesthesiologist as soon as possible.
- Tell the anesthesiologist in advance that you prefer not to receive a transfusion before surgery.
- Ask: Is PCA available for postoperative pain relief?

For liver transplants:

- If your friend or family member is waiting for a liver transplant, accompany him or her to the preoperative consultation with the anesthesiologist and bring all pertinent medical information.
- If the patient seems to be in pain after surgery, or you notice that the patient is bleeding, is not breathing properly, has a decreased level of consciousness, or is confused, notify the nurse.

CHAPTER 12

. . .

Orthopedic Surgery

. . .

Tricia, a sixty-two-year-old woman with rheumatoid arthritis, was scheduled for a hip replacement. A week before her surgery, she came to our preoperative anesthesia clinic, bringing with her a list of the medications she'd been taking. These included nonsteroidal anti-inflammatory drugs (NSAIDs)—she found ibuprofen particularly effective—as well as steroids prescribed to relieve pain.

Among other information, Tricia told the anesthesiologist who saw her that the last time she'd had surgery, the anesthesiologist had had trouble inserting the breathing tube. Arthritis causes the neck to become rigid, so we can't manipulate the patient's head as usual to place the tube. It was fortunate that Tricia mentioned this, since it prepared the anesthesiologist to expect the same problem when she had to intubate Tricia.

Next, Tricia asked to have epidural anesthesia, and the anesthesiologist agreed, adding that the epidural could be used as well for postoperative pain relief. She also instructed Tricia to stop taking ibuprofen during the remaining days before surgery, and to switch instead to Tylenol or another form of acetaminophen, explaining that this was the only type of NSAID that did not interfere with blood clotting. (This instruction is standard practice in some hospitals but not in all, since there is disagreement about whether taking these drugs causes excess bleeding during surgery.)

The following week, Tricia arrived for surgery as a same-day-admit patient. Questioning her just before the procedure, the anesthesiologist discovered that, since Tricia had thought she wasn't supposed to take anything by mouth right before surgery, she hadn't had her dose of steroid that morning. The anesthesiologist therefore administered it right after inserting the IV line, to prevent Tricia from experiencing withdrawal—in the form of life-threatening hypotension—during the procedure. The anesthesiologist then gave her an epidural, and the staff placed her on the table, positioning her lying on one side to give the surgeon access to the opposite hip.

Immediately, Tricia complained that this position was causing pain in her other joints. The anesthesiologist administered sedation and analgesia, but the pain continued to bother her so much that the anesthesiologist was ultimately forced to give her general anesthesia—which turned out to be quite difficult, just as expected. After some effort the anesthesiologist was able to intubate her using a fiberoptic laryngoscope, and the surgery could continue.

Tricia's experience illustrates the kind of trade-off decisions we must often make when deciding what type of anesthesia to give older patients having orthopedic surgery. Although theoretically, giving Tricia regional anesthesia was a good idea, considering her condition and her history it would actually have been better to give her both a regional and a general at the outset. That way, her airway would have been taken care of early on, without having to interrupt the surgery, and an epidural would still be in place for pain relief both during and after the operation.

Tricia did make a good recovery, demonstrating the value of the continuous epidural in allowing early movement. The morning after surgery, she was able to sit on the side of the bed and move her feet. That afternoon, she walked fairly comfortably with a walker. And since she was up and about so soon, the risk of deep vein thrombosis and pneumonia was minimized.

Challenges of Orthopedic Surgery

Orthopedic procedures are among the most common types of surgery performed today. In addition to arthritis, we do them for congenital anomalies, sports injuries, and other types of accidents. For both the anesthesiologist and the patient, however, these procedures can be challenging. Although they lend themselves to the use of regional anesthesia, sudden difficulties can crop up, as we saw with Tricia.

A number of other problems can make managing anesthesia for orthopedic surgery difficult. To perform the different procedures, we must place the patient in a variety of awkward positions whose discomfort may make general anesthesia necessary, as happened with Tricia. Because patients with arthritis have usually been quite inactive, they are particularly prone to develop deep vein thrombosis, so that a pulmonary embolism can occur, often three to four days after surgery. What's more, when long bones have been fractured, or a hip is being replaced, emboli composed of fat particles from inside the bones can also enter the blood, traveling to the lungs and potentially to the brain, where they can block circulation.

During orthopedic surgery, patients commonly lose a great deal of blood, so for these procedures it's particularly important to be able to reinfuse their own blood. One technique for doing this is autologous blood transfusion. Two weeks before surgery, your own blood is drawn and stored so it can be used during the operation. During those two weeks, the body replenishes the blood to near normal levels. If anticipated blood loss is great, a cell saver should also be used during surgery to salvage your blood for retransfusion should this be necessary.

The following discussion is organized by parts of the body instead of by disorders, since anesthetic management is similar for sports injuries; degenerative diseases, such as arthritis; and accidents. There is a difference, however, between elderly and younger patients. Elderly people often have chronic lung disease, hypertension, coronary artery disease, rheumatoid arthritis, and possibly impaired blood coagulation resulting from the use of NSAIDs to control arthritic pain. Accident victims and people with sports injuries, by contrast, are usually young and healthy, so they don't experience the medical complications we see in older people. Anesthesia for young people tends to be less complicated, and they have more choices regarding the type of anesthesia to have. Unlike Tricia, a young man who breaks his hip in a football game, for example, usually doesn't have arthritis; he can be sedated and receive regional anesthesia without experiencing pain from other joints while lying on the table.

The operations described below are performed as either ambulatory or inpatient procedures, depending on their complexity, the potential for postoperative complications, and the patient's preexisting medical conditions.

Shoulder Injuries

Operations are usually performed on the shoulder after dislocations, injuries of the rotator cuff (the tough band of tendon and muscle around the shoulder joint), and fractures. Anesthesia can be either regional or general.

Regional anesthesia for a shoulder procedure consists of an upper extremity block (which affects the arm on the involved side). The nerves that supply the shoulder pass out of the spinal cord at discrete locations, so it's relatively easy to block them with local anesthetics. We also place a continuous catheter at the base of the neck in front, so that if the procedure is lengthy, we can reinject the anesthetic when it wears off. The catheter also provides postoperative pain relief until the patient is discharged. For those who stay in the hospital as inpatients, the catheter can be left in place for up to three days. It works like a continuous epidural and can be patient-controlled; when pain returns, you simply inject more of the drug.

Before placing the catheter or administering the block, however, the anesthesiologist must do an extensive examination to search for existing nerve injury. She or he looks for numbness around the shoulder or arm or a limitation in movement of the arm or shoulder. Any impairment must be clearly documented so that, after the operation, the anesthesia will not be suspected of causing neurologic injury (which is a remote possibility).

A shoulder procedure requires the patient to remain motionless in a rather uncomfortable semisitting position with the affected shoulder and arm extended outward. For young, healthy people we can administer sedation and analgesia to make it less uncomfortable without having to worry that it will depress their breathing. With the elderly, however, we have to be concerned that the sedative will depress respiration (see chapter 7 for an explanation of why this happens), so they may need general anesthesia. Younger people who don't want a regional can also have general anesthesia.

Elbow, Wrist, and Hand Surgery

For operations on the elbow, wrist, and hand, we prefer regional anesthesia, which consists of a brachial block (affecting the brachial plexus, a network of nerves in the neck) placed above the collarbone. An axillary block placed in the armpit is an alternative, preferred by some doctors to avoid pneumothorax (accumulation of air in the chest that compresses the lungs, preventing them from expanding). Again, we can leave a catheter in place for long procedures and for pain control afterward. If the patient wishes, we can also perform these operations under general anesthesia.

Carpal tunnel syndrome has grown more widespread in recent years due to the increased use of computers. This condition can arise from fibrosis (formation of tough, fibrous tissue) around tendons that enable the hands to move. (The carpal tunnel is a passage inside the wrist through which run these tendons and the median nerve; pressure on this nerve from the fibrosed tendons causes the pain.) The syndrome results from chronic strain following long periods of repetitive movement, such as performed by assembly-line workers or computer keyboarders. Carpal tunnel syndrome not only decreases hand movement but causes pain that often becomes severe enough to make sufferers unable to work.

The condition should not be treated surgically until more conservative treatments—such as rest, physical therapy, and ergonomic adjustment of work habits and equipment—have failed. This is because surgery does not always work; often the pain recurs. The surgeon removes the fibrous tissue, releasing the tendons to allow pain-free movement. Since the fibrous tissue can and does return over time, physical therapy is mandatory after the operation to decrease the likelihood of recurrence.

For this operation we give regional anesthesia, generally with an axillary block, although some surgeons prefer to inject the area with local anesthetics. In my opinion, this is probably not a good choice, since frequently a tourniquet is placed around the upper arm during the procedure to decrease bleeding. If you haven't had the axillary block, the tourniquet can be painful.

- Request an axillary block during surgery for carpal tunnel syndrome.

Hip Surgery

Fractures, degenerative arthritis, and congenital abnormalities including dislocations (which are surgically corrected in children and also sometimes in adults) are all reasons why people have hip replacement surgery. Here again, if patients are young, the procedure is relatively easy, while if they're elderly, it's more complicated. Since many people who have hip replacements are elderly, medical management of preexisting diseases is usually necessary.

- Be sure to take a list of all the medical conditions you're being treated for, as well as all the medications you're taking, to the preoperative consultation.

Hip surgery tends to be uncomfortable, as Tricia learned. To make matters worse, we often use a specialized table called a "fracture table" to allow appropriate positioning; this table is completely flat, without any breaking points, so it can't be adjusted to make you more comfortable. Even a young patient with no diseases is likely to experience extreme discomfort during a hip replacement, which is why young as well as old may want general anesthesia for this procedure. Elderly people, moreover, often

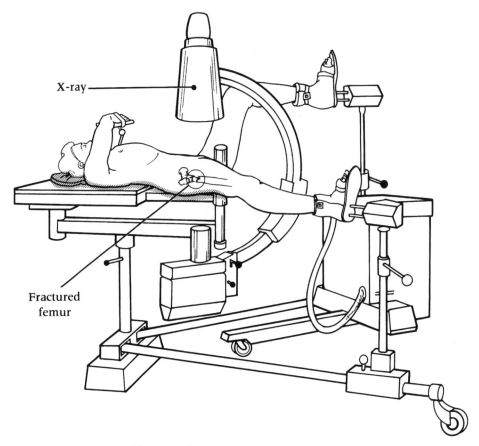

X-ray

Fractured
femur

Fig. 15. Fracture table for hip fracture repair. Once the patient is in position, the bottom half of the table is removed.

have sensitive skin, especially if they have arthritis or have been treated with steroids, and are prone to developing ulcers when lying motionless for a long period.

- If your skin is sensitive, make sure the anesthesiologist knows to place appropriate padding under areas that will be subject to pressure.
- If you have a preference for being awake or asleep, let the anesthesiologist know. If you want to be asleep, you can still have a regional for postoperative pain control.

There is considerable blood loss during a hip replacement, so you will need either cell salvaging or autologous blood transfusion.

- Ask the anesthesiologist whether cell salvaging is available or if it's possible to do autologous blood transfusion, so you can avoid the possible complications of regular transfusion, especially infection with hepatitis C or HIV.

To minimize blood loss, the anesthesiologist may use a special procedure called deliberate hypotension. We give a vasodilator drug like nitroprusside to reduce your blood pressure to a minimal yet safe level, monitoring it closely with an arterial catheter. The anesthesiologist must determine exactly what this minimal blood pressure level is for each patient. In someone with untreated high blood pressure, for example, the level must be higher than for someone who has normal blood pressure or someone who has high blood pressure that has been treated. Deliberate hypotension can actually decrease your need for blood transfusion.

- Ask if it's possible to prevent bleeding during surgery by reducing blood pressure, as long as you have no medical contraindications.

If you have coronary artery disease or have been treated for transient ischemic attack (temporary interruption of blood flow to the brain, causing strokelike symptoms) or stroke, reducing your blood pressure could trigger a heart attack or another stroke.

While inducing deliberate hypotension, the anesthesiologist must take into account still another factor affecting blood pressure. In inserting the artificial joint, the surgeon uses a special glue to attach the ball that replaces the head of the thigh bone to the shaft of the bone. This glue is absorbed into the bloodstream and depresses heart function, causing hypotension. The anesthesiologist must be particularly alert when the patient has preexisting coronary artery disease or stroke; if blood pressure gets too low, he or she raises it by immediately administering vasopressors.

Knee Surgery

With fitness an increasing obsession—especially among the baby boomers—knee surgery has been on the rise, for all that extra physical exertion tends to wear out the joints. Thus more and more people are having procedures called arthroscopies ("arthro" derives from the Greek word for joint) to diagnose knee disorders. Arthroscopy and the other procedures described in this section are generally performed in ambulatory surgery units.

For an arthroscopy, a small incision is made around the knee, and a fiberoptic scope with a light source is inserted to visualize the interior of the joint. To make viewing easier, fluid is infused into the knee, which can accumulate and increase the amount of pain the patient feels during the procedure. Usually, the surgeon is looking for a damaged ligament or meniscus (one of two crescent-shaped structures made of cartilage that act as cushions between the bones of the knee).

Depending on what the problem is, the surgeon may be able to treat it surgically on the spot, through the arthroscope. Otherwise you may need open surgery on the knee.

Since arthroscopy and open knee surgery are most often done for healthy adults and require less positioning than hip surgery, these procedures are usually performed under regional anesthesia. Generally, this means a spinal, but if the surgeon thinks the operation will be complicated, an epidural might be a better choice. With an epidural the anesthetic can be reinjected if the procedure takes a long time (spinals are not repeated because the patient can't be repositioned to allow another shot to be placed). Also, before the patient is discharged, we can give a final dose of narcotic through the epidural catheter that will provide pain control through the night.

Sometimes regional anesthesia is contraindicated. There may be infection in the area where the spinal or epidural would be placed, or the patient has had previous back surgery that fused the vertebrae in that area, making it too difficult to place a needle there. In such cases we use specific nerve blocks. To ensure complete pain relief, we need to block multiple nerves.

Knee replacements are more complicated than arthroscopies or even open knee surgery to repair torn tissues. Because replacements take much longer, I recommend either epidural or general anesthesia. In these procedures, a tourniquet is usually applied just above the knee to decrease bleeding. It may cause pain, which can be relieved by deflating the tourniquet for a few minutes during the procedure. Deflation of the tourniquet at the end of the operation may result in hypotension due to the presence of toxic substances that accumulated in the leg while no blood was flowing through it. The anesthesiologist must be prepared to treat this hypotension by rapidly infusing fluids and/or vasopressors.

- If you're having any knee procedure, request spinal anesthesia if the surgeon thinks the procedure will be short and uncomplicated.
- If the procedure will be more complex, ask for an epidural with a final injection before the catheter is removed, for postoperative pain relief.

Ankle Surgery

Surgery is performed less often on the ankles than on the knees; usually it's for traumatic injuries. Diagnosis is by x-ray, and treatment is usually by open surgery. Anesthesia is the same as for knee surgery. If you have specific nerve blocks, however, five are needed, although these are more easily placed because the nerves in question are more accessible. If you prefer not to have a spinal or epidural because you don't want a needle in your back, you can request a regional.

Bunionectomy

A bunion is a deformity of the big toe that results from degenerative arthritis or injury. It is painful and prevents you from wearing shoes. Bunions are removed in a procedure called bunionectomy, which is usually done under regional anesthesia since it involves resecting actual bone, which is painful. It's possible to place ankle blocks instead, but these would not prevent possible pain from a tourniquet that is applied above the knee to prevent bleeding. Therefore, I suggest that you request a spinal for this procedure. If you have any deformities of the spine that preclude a spinal, I recommend a combined block of the femoral and sciatic nerves. If you don't want to be awake, you can also have general anesthesia.

- If you're having a bunion removed, ask for a spinal or, if you prefer not to be awake, general anesthesia.

Microvascular Surgery

Surgery performed under a microscope can replace fingers, toes, arms, hands, legs, and feet that have been accidentally amputated. These microvascular techniques for reattaching tiny blood vessels, nerves, and ligaments have made it possible for severed limbs to function almost normally after surgery.

As you might expect, these procedures are long—lasting twenty-four or even thirty-six hours, which means another surgical team must be available to replace the surgeon and anesthesiologist at intervals. Since an awake patient is generally unable to lie on the operating table for this length of time, microvascular surgery normally involves general anesthesia. For the anesthesiologist, such a procedure poses unique problems. First, we need to maintain the patient's body temperature, since under general anesthesia, people lose the ability to do this themselves. Unless external heating is applied, the body tends to come to room temperature, and operating rooms are generally kept colder than normal rooms because surgeons wear multiple layers of gowns for the sake of sterility and infection control. Thus we warm the patient with blankets heated by warm air.

Second, it's critical to maximize the blood flow to the reattached limb. We do this by giving inhalation anesthetics to relax and open the blood vessels and sometimes also by giving local anesthetics to block the sympathetic nerves (which contract the blood vessels). At the same time, we prevent clotting in the newly attached limb by administering fluids that will decrease the viscosity of the blood.

Postoperatively, it's essential that the patient stay warm and free from anxiety. If you become cold or anxious, your body releases hormones that cause the blood vessels to contract and thus put your reimplanted limb at risk for tissue death.

Degenerative Diseases of the Spine

A number of degenerative conditions can make the spine unstable, disrupting the normal alignment of the vertebrae and leading to a deformity that winds up injuring the spinal cord or the major nerve roots leading out of it. This instability must be corrected as soon as possible to prevent further neurological damage.

One such condition is "slipped disk," in which one of the elastic disks that provide cushioning between the vertebrae protrudes out of place and compresses the spinal cord or nerve roots. Another is osteoarthritis, a noninflammatory degenerative disease of the joints that causes abnormal bone growth and development of bony spurs on the edges of the vertebrae, which press on the nerves. Spinal stenosis is a congenital condition in which there is too little space within the spinal canal for the nerves passing through it; symptoms may not appear until adulthood. Spondylolysis and spondylolisthesis both involve defects in a vertebra, sometimes congenital and sometimes caused by injury or degenerative disease, which cause it to slip forward over the vertebra beneath. The result can be severe pain and nerve injury. Finally, degenerative diseases such as ankylosing spondylitis and rheumatoid arthritis can make the spine completely rigid.

Patients with these conditions need extensive surgery to stabilize the vertebrae at different levels of the spine. These procedures carry risks of large amounts of blood loss, of paralysis, and of venous air embolism, in which blood passing through veins in the vertebrae sucks in air that is carried to the heart, lungs, or brain, decreasing oxygenation.

Preoperative Consultation

For procedures on the spine, a preoperative consultation with your anesthesiologist is an absolute necessity. The anesthesiologist must pay particular attention to deformities in the cervical spine (of the neck) and the throat that might interfere with managing your airway during surgery. This is critically important, since the patient generally lies face down, so the airway isn't accessible.

Frequently, patients who need this type of surgery must be intubated with a fiberoptic laryngoscope. Usually, they are older and have other medical conditions, such as hypertension and impaired kidney function. We must bring hypertension under control before they can have surgery and must give special drugs both during and after the operation to treat the increases in blood pressure that may develop. Because such people are generally taking numerous drugs, the anesthesiologist needs accurate information about current medications.

- Bring a list of all the drugs you're taking to the preoperative consultation.
- Tell the anesthesiologist if you have any limitation of movement in your neck or any pain on moving your head.

Anesthesia for Surgery

Surgery on the spine is generally done under general anesthesia since the deformities in an unstable spine may make it difficult to place a regional, and attempting to do so can—in rare cases—worsen the patient's neurological symptoms. Although some anesthesiologists have administered regional anesthesia successfully in such cases, I prefer to give general anesthesia for all types of surgery for extensive degenerative spinal diseases. Either an epidural or a spinal is satisfactory for brief procedures, such as laminectomy (removal of a lamina, part of the bony arch of a vertebra that encloses the spinal cord) or diskectomy (removal of an intervertebral disk).

- If your anesthesiologist intends to give you regional anesthesia for spinal surgery, ask how long the surgery will last and whether you would be more comfortable in the prone position under general anesthesia.

For these procedures we may use evoked potentials to monitor spinal cord function. Sometimes we must also do wake-up testing to check the patient's ability to move: we stop the anesthetic and ask you to move your arms or legs to be sure there's been no damage to the cord that's causing paralysis. To make wake-up possible, we use anesthetics such as propofol that wear off rapidly, while at the same time allowing narcotics—which don't prevent movement—to stay on board so you can move the arm or leg but without feeling any pain.

The complexity of the anesthetic management depends on what level of the spine is being operated on: cervical (neck), thoracic (chest), or lumbar (low back). The cervical area is the most difficult, since the anesthesiologist has to manage the airway without causing movement of the cervical spine that could further damage the spinal cord. To make intubation possible, we use specialized techniques to apply local anesthesia to the upper part of the airway: nerve blocks in the neck and inhalation of vaporized local anesthetics, often accompanied by sedation.

When the cervical spine is very unstable, we perform fiberoptic intubation. Generally, we keep the patients awake and perform the intubation as they lie on their back on a stretcher. If the surgery will be performed in the prone position, once the tube is in place, we ask them to turn over onto the operating table on their stomach; the ability to do this demonstrates that the cord hasn't been injured. Now the evoked potentials monitor is placed, and then we give general anesthesia.

Surgery on the thoracic and lumbar spine is no less complicated, but anesthesia induction is easier, since these precautions aren't necessary.

Postoperative Pain Control

Since most spine surgery is done under general anesthesia, postoperative pain control is largely by patient-controlled analgesia, which provides better relief than intramuscular injection of narcotics. At the end of the operation, the surgeon may inject local anesthetics or narcotics, which will last about four hours; when they wear off you receive PCA through a catheter in the back of your hand.

Postoperatively, we observe you for weakness or limitation of movement in the arms and/or legs, depending on the level of the surgery. After cervical surgery, for example, we check for decreased movement or paralysis in all four limbs. After lumbar or thoracic surgery, we observe the legs and check for possible difficulty in urinating.

- If your arms or legs feel weak, or you have difficulty urinating, notify the surgeon immediately.

Anesthesia in the Cast Room

The cast room in the hospital is where fractures are set, casts and bandages changed, pins removed, dislocated hips and shoulders relocated, and joints manipulated to increase their range of motion after cast removal. Since all these procedures can be extremely painful, they require anesthesia.

Many patients who have these procedures come in as emergencies, and therefore present a variety of challenges to the anesthesiologist. Often they have full stomachs, which means a risk of aspirating stomach contents into the lungs. Similarly, accidents frequently happen to people who have gone to parties and used alcohol or recreational drugs. Minor procedures are usually done under conscious sedation administered by the surgeon, without an anesthesiologist present. For more complex procedures, regional anesthesia is best, since it minimizes the risk that someone who has just eaten will aspirate stomach contents into the lungs, as well as the risk that someone with alcohol or other drugs in his or her system will be oversedated, which would cause respiratory depression (see chapter 2 on the risks of aspiration and chapter 5 for a description of the risks for anesthesia posed by drugs and alcohol).

In administering a regional, the anesthesiologist must choose a local anesthetic that will provide anesthesia only for the duration of the procedure and not last for a long time afterward. This prevents you from injuring the part that's anesthetized and can't feel. If you fractured your wrist, for example, and had a regional, your entire arm would be numb, and if you touched a hot object you'd be burned because you couldn't feel the heat.

- If you receive a spinal or epidural, make sure you can urinate on your own before you go home. Otherwise, you might have to return to have a catheter placed to empty your bladder.

- After the surgery, ask how long your arm or leg will stay numb.

You'll need to remain particularly alert during this period, to prevent injury. If you've had a long-acting anesthetic, you might have to watch yourself for as long as ten hours. If you can, have someone around to watch what your arm or leg comes in contact with—if your finger got caught in a door, you might not notice it until after the damage had been done.

Summary: Questions and Points to Remember

General Questions about Orthopedic Procedures

- Decide whether or not you'd feel comfortable receiving regional anesthesia.

This decision can be based on your anxiety level in response to the thought of being awake while you're pushed and pulled around. Remember too that you'll have to remain almost motionless in a strange position on the operating table during the procedure.

- During the preoperative consultation, ask whether cell salvaging can be used during your operation.
- Ask if you can donate blood to be used in case you need it during the procedure.
- If you have general anesthesia, request in addition a regional anesthetic with a continuous catheter to be used primarily for postoperative pain relief.
- If you don't have a regional, remember that you will have more pain after the operation when it's necessary to begin moving about—and that if you don't move, you could develop deep vein thrombosis and possibly a pulmonary embolism.
- If you are elderly and have a condition such as osteoarthritis or rheumatoid arthritis that affects most of your joints, don't hesitate to request general anesthesia.

Without general anesthesia, you could become extremely uncomfortable during the operation. Remember that you can have a regional too, administered after general anesthesia has been induced, for postoperative pain relief.

- Although some experts don't think this is necessary, I recommend that you avoid taking ibuprofen and aspirin for two weeks before your surgery; it's OK to take acetaminophen.

Remember that blood coagulation is critical during orthopedic procedures and that taking these drugs may impair it.

- If you have taken these drugs within two weeks of surgery, be sure to tell the anesthesiologist, because surgery may have to be postponed. If it's an emergency, steps can be taken to minimize bleeding.

Specific Procedures

- Request an axillary block during surgery for carpal tunnel syndrome.

When having hip surgery:

- Be sure to take a list of all the medical conditions you're being treated for, as well as all the medications you're taking, to the preoperative consultation.
- If your skin is sensitive, make sure the anesthesiologist knows to place appropriate padding under areas that will be subject to pressure.
- If you have a preference for being awake or asleep, let the anesthesiologist know. If you want to be asleep, you can still have a regional for postoperative pain control.
- Ask the anesthesiologist whether cell salvaging is available or if it's possible to do autologous blood transfusion, so you can avoid the possible complications of regular transfusion, especially infection with hepatitis C or HIV.
- Ask if it's possible to prevent bleeding during surgery by reducing blood pressure, as long as you have no medical contraindications.

For knee surgery:

- If you're having any knee procedure, request spinal anesthesia if the surgeon thinks the procedure will be short and uncomplicated.
- If the procedure will be more complex, ask for an epidural with a final injection before the catheter is removed, for postoperative pain relief.

For bunionectomy:

- If you're having a bunion removed, ask for a spinal or, if you prefer not to be awake, general anesthesia.

For procedures on the spine:

- Bring a list of all the drugs you're taking to the preoperative consultation.
- Tell the anesthesiologist if you have any limitation of movement in your neck or any pain on moving your head.
- If your anesthesiologist intends to give you regional anesthesia for spinal surgery, ask how long the surgery will last and whether you would be more comfortable in the prone position under general anesthesia.
- After surgery, if your arms or legs feel weak, or you have difficulty urinating, notify the surgeon immediately.

For procedures in the cast room:

- If you receive a spinal or epidural, make sure you can urinate on your own before you go home.
- After the surgery, ask how long your arm or leg will stay numb.

CHAPTER 13

• • •

Urinary Conditions

• • •

On the night before Robert Lipsyte, *New York Times* columnist and author, was scheduled for a long, complicated operation for testicular cancer, his anesthesiologist dropped in for a preoperative visit. Explaining at great length how important the anesthesia was, she assured Lipsyte that if he were to die, it would be due to the anesthesia, not the surgery. "Hearing this just before a radical operation scared the shit out of me," Lipsyte recalled.

"The next morning in the OR, just as I was sliding under, this same anesthesiologist, who was chattering to the other OR staff about her recent vacation, as an afterthought leaned close to me and whispered in my ear, 'Don't worry about a thing. Dr. R— will have no trouble removing your prostate.' As I tried to object that my prostate wasn't the part in question, I slowly lost consciousness. But I remembered the overwhelming anxiety of trying to object and being unable to. Fortunately the surgeon did know which organ to remove!"

Afterward, Lipsyte went on, "I felt like I was coming back from two separate things: it seemed that I recovered from the surgery more quickly than from the anesthesia. My brain was fuzzy. In fact it was a month before I regained the complete mental clarity I had before the operation."

In his 1998 book *In the Country of Illness: Comfort and Advice for the Journey*, Lipsyte describes his experience of cancer as a voyage into what he calls the country of "Malady,"which included an education in the native customs of medical personnel. As one of these natives, I can tell you that anesthesiologists often forget how worried people are when they're brought into the operating room. We need to take care not to have conversations with other staff members before the patient is asleep. I generally ask that the staff not talk except to answer questions from the patient or to request needed equipment until the patient is safely asleep.

People about to have surgery on their urinary tract are particularly worried. Their sense of modesty is injured by the need to expose such a

private area; they feel shy, and are also possessed by anxiety over potential sexual dysfunction. Surgery on the urinary tract is an especially delicate prospect because of all the connotations associated with this part of
the body. One of the best ways to cope, then, is to understand exactly
what is going to happen and what your options are, so you can be better
in control.

Diagnostic and Treatment Techniques

Most diagnostic and surgical procedures for treating disorders of the urinary tract are noninvasive; they're done endoscopically (using a tubular
instrument that allows visualization of the interior of an organ), through
a catheter inserted through the urethra and into the bladder. For simpler
procedures, the tube is usually a rigid *cystoscope* with a light at the end.
The surgeon can look through the scope directly into the bladder. More
complicated procedures may require a flexible *fiberoptic scope*, which
enables the surgeon to visualize the organs indirectly on a video screen.
Through these instruments we can diagnose and also treat conditions such
as kidney stones, blockages of the ureters (the tubes that carry urine from
the kidneys to the bladder), and tumors of the bladder or prostate.

Another diagnostic technique is *laparoscopic surgery*. A tube is inserted
through an incision in the abdomen to look for enlarged lymph nodes,
which could indicate a serious problem, such as metastatic carcinoma of
the urinary system, lymphoma, or a severe infection. To improve visibility we infuse air into the abdominal cavity to make the abdominal wall
stand away from the organs. This procedure, which can cause cramping,
requires either general or regional anesthesia.

Many urological problems are treated endoscopically by laser surgery
or electrocautery. *Laser surgery* can remove warts on the external geni-
tals as well as small tumors throughout the urinary system. It tends to be
less painful than other types of surgery and to cause less bleeding. Often
the patient needs only sedation and analgesia, sometimes assisted with
local anesthesia.

In *electrocautery* an electric current runs through a wire loop that's used
to cut and burn tissue. We use electrocautery to resect bladder tumors and
benign enlargements of the prostate gland. Because it generates heat, electrocautery is more painful than a laser, so you need more anesthesia.

Many surgical procedures on the urinary system are performed for
people at the extremes of age: children and those over sixty-five. Therefore in addition to the considerations described in this chapter, the special

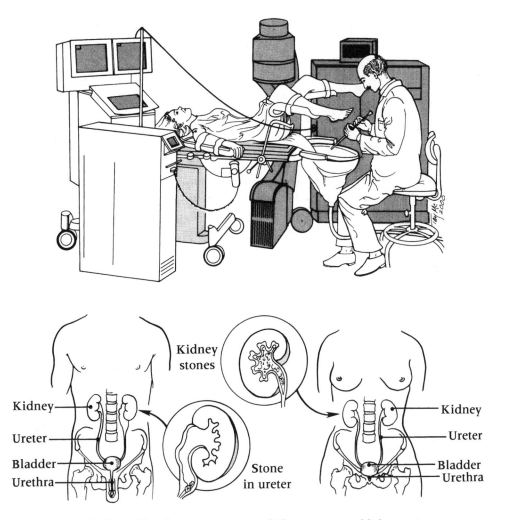

Fig. 16. Male and female urinary systems, kidney stones, and lithotripsy machine with physician performing cystoscopy.

anesthetic requirements of these two groups, as explained in chapter 7, must be taken into account.

Procedures on the Bladder

Procedures performed to diagnose and treat carcinoma of the bladder, to treat strictures of the bladder neck (narrowing caused by previous infection or injury), and to assess infection are the most frequent types of urinary tract surgery. Also common are procedures for diagnosing and treating bladder prolapse in women; these are described in chapter 6.

The anesthesia required for bladder procedures ranges from simple sedation and analgesia to complete general anesthesia and/or regional anesthesia. A woman having a cystoscopy—a diagnostic procedure in which the cystoscope is passed through the urethra into the bladder—may need only sedation and analgesia, supplied by the anesthesiologist, along with a local anesthetic in the form of a jelly applied to the scope by the urologist. For a man, cystoscopy is more painful because the urethra is longer, so we generally prefer regional or even general anesthesia.

Bladder Tumor Resection

Bladder tumors are removed endoscopically, either by a laser or by electrocautery. If there are only one or two areas of tumor in the bladder, the procedure can be done under sedation and analgesia. Extensive bladder tumors, however, require more anesthesia. They are best performed under spinal rather than general anesthesia, because fluids are infused to wash away blood and tumor fragments as the resection proceeds. Since this fluid is infused under pressure, and since veins in the area are open, the body can absorb it. Excess fluid absorption can cause various complications that the anesthesiologist must be alert to avoid: congestive heart failure from fluid overload, brain edema (swelling that results from imbalance in blood electrolytes), and pulmonary edema (excess fluid in the lungs).

If you remain awake during this procedure, the anesthesiologist can watch you for signs of abnormal brain function, such as confusion or agitation. We can also see whether you're breathing normally and catch any signs of respiratory distress. Then we can treat you early before significant damage occurs in your brain, heart, or lungs. If you insist on general anesthesia, on the other hand, we can't monitor for these indications as easily, making it much more difficult to diagnose problems while they're still developing. So the safest type of anesthesia to have for resection of a bladder tumor (and for removal of a prostate tumor; see the descriptions of prostate resection below) is regional.

- If you're having an extensive bladder tumor removed, request spinal anesthesia—no matter how afraid of it you may be—to reduce the risk of a serious complication.

During bladder tumor resection, the anesthesiologist must be alert to three other possible problems: hypothermia, blood loss, and coagulation abnormalities. As you can imagine, the combination of major blood loss and blood that doesn't clot can create serious problems.

Hypothermia (low body temperature) occurs because the fluid being infused is at room temperature, whereas normal body temperature is much higher. Since the bladder is very vascular (richly supplied with blood vessels), whenever part of it is removed, we see major blood loss. Abnormal blood coagulation results both because clotting factors in the blood are diluted by the extra fluid being infused and because of hypothermia, since when the body temperature drops, certain clotting factors aren't produced. The anesthesiologist therefore keeps body temperature normal with a warming blanket, a device resembling an air mattress through which blows a constant flow of warm air, while a temperature monitor maintains a constant temperature.

Procedures on the Ureters

To diagnose obstructions of the ureter caused by infection, kidney stones, or tumors, a catheter or an endoscope is threaded through the bladder and up into the ureter itself. Procedures on the ureters are often quite painful, and you may need regional or even general anesthesia.

Once the obstruction is diagnosed, the patient may have an endoscopic procedure called percutaneous nephrostomy. We insert a scope through an incision in the flank and introduce a catheter into the kidney to bypass the obstruction so that the urine can flow to the outside of the body, where it's collected in a bag. This is a temporary measure until definitive surgery can be performed to remove the obstruction.

Since no air is infused, and the instrument enters the ureter from the side instead of passing up through its length, this procedure is less painful and requires less anesthesia. The patient usually lies face down while the anesthesiologist administers sedation and analgesia and the surgeon administers a local anesthetic.

Lithotripsy for Kidney Stones

Kidney stones are usually treated with scopes through which the surgeon passes tiny instruments that catch the stones and pull them out of the urethra or bladder. Stones that are too large to be removed this way are crushed by a procedure called lithotripsy, which uses focused sound waves.

Anesthesia for lithotripsy can be challenging, depending on how the procedure is performed, for there are two generations of equipment in use. In order to generate the sound waves that are focused on the stone, the older lithotripsy machines require that the patient sit up in a chair in a tub of water. Immersed in water in an uncomfortable position, the patient is often quite anxious, so the anesthesiologist must sedate him or her enough to prevent any movement during the procedure. This means balancing the dose of sedative against the possibility of overdosing and causing respiratory depression.

We can also give regional anesthesia, but both types of regional create their own problems. Giving an epidural means leaving a catheter in place, which requires special precautions to prevent infection from the contaminated water. We could give a spinal before placing the patient in the water, but this would make the patient unable to use his or her legs, making it quite difficult to seat the patient in the chair. And if we give a general, the entire body has to be supported during transfer into the tub.

We also prefer conscious sedation because it leaves the patient feeling comfortable and untroubled, yet still able to respond to commands, such as being asked to breathe deeply. What's more, lithotripsy is often performed at a distance from the operating room, which means that few anesthesia personnel are around to assist if complications occur. Thus the procedure is much safer if you're able to cooperate and stay in verbal contact with the anesthesiologist.

These problems don't arise with the newer generation of lithotripsy equipment, since these machines don't require immersion in water. Instead they use a water-filled cushion placed against the patient's flank. Accordingly, anesthesia is easier, and we don't need to worry about keeping you awake. Although sedation and analgesia are commonly used, it's fine to request general anesthesia if you prefer it. Regional anesthesia—either spinal or epidural—is also safe, although a spinal may be preferable because it can be placed more quickly. Besides, since there's often no need for postoperative pain relief, you don't need an epidural catheter in place.

Prostate Surgery

Cancer and benign enlargement of the prostate gland are diagnosed with a fiberoptic scope, a digital rectal exam, and a blood test. If carcinoma is suspected, a biopsy is taken through the rectum, usually under conscious sedation. Surgery to relieve the obstruction of urine flow caused by the tumor or benign enlargement is also done through a scope.

The possible complications here are the same as for resection of bladder tumors: again, the enlargement or tumor is resected bit by bit, with tumor fragments and blood washed away by fluid irrigation, so the anesthesiologist must watch for brain, heart, and lung abnormalities indicating fluid absorption and overload. As with bladder tumor resection, therefore, regional anesthesia is preferable since it gives us the best chance to detect any complications as they develop. Since here too there's a risk of blood loss, we may ask patients to donate their blood two weeks in advance, so it can be given to them during or after their surgery; this is known as autologous blood transfusion.

Open Surgical Procedures

Complete removal of the bladder or prostate gland, as well as surgery to remove kidney tumors, can't be done through a scope but requires open surgery.

Radical Prostatectomy

In a radical prostatectomy, the entire prostate gland is removed. This operation requires general anesthesia; often we give a regional as well, especially an epidural for postoperative pain relief. Radical prostatectomy involves significant blood loss, so if possible we use a central venous pressure catheter to determine when transfusion is needed. For most patients we recommend predonation of blood two weeks ahead of time so they can have an autologous blood transfusion.

The operation is performed with the patient in a supine position, lying on his back with legs spread and pelvis tilted forward by a bend in the operating room table. This position puts considerable stress on the low back, and patients often complain of low back pain that lasts about a week after surgery. Many assume that this was caused by the epidural, but in fact that's not the case.

I once managed the anesthesia for two radical prostatectomies within a two-week period. Mark was seventy-eight and had numerous other medical conditions, as such patients often do. He had had a heart attack and an angioplasty, was being treated for high blood pressure, and was a social drinker. Matthew was forty-six and in relatively good health. Both had the same anesthesia—a general plus an epidural, though Matthew was reluctant to accept the epidural because he didn't want a needle in his back. I had to work hard to convince him that it was the best option to relieve postoperative pain and prevent deep vein thrombosis by enabling him to walk right after surgery.

Both surgeries went well, but afterward Matthew complained of severe lower back pain, which he insisted was the result of the epidural. I tried to convince him otherwise, but it was impossible. Mark, on the other hand, was pain-free during most of his postoperative period and went home without complaints. There is simply no explanation for this difference in outcomes.

- During the preoperative consultation with your anesthesiologist, ask for an epidural, which can be used for postoperative pain control. If you have serious objections to having an epidural for a radical prostatectomy, you can simply refuse—but I don't recommend that you do.
- Ask to donate your blood in advance so it's available for autologous transfusion.

Orchiectomy

Orchiectomy, the removal of one or both testicles, is performed after traumatic injuries, to resect carcinomas, and to treat prostate cancer. Most often, it is performed under spinal anesthesia; but if you prefer, you can have general.

Procedures on the Scrotum

Spermatocelectomy is excision of a spermatocele, a tumorlike mass composed of sperm seminal fluid that builds up in the scrotum. *Varicocelectomy* is excision of a collection of enlarged veins in the scrotum; the veins are resected just like varicose veins in the leg. Both procedures are performed to relieve pain and to reverse infertility. They're done under spinal, epidural, or general anesthesia, depending on the patient's, surgeon's, and anesthesiologist's choices.

Complete Bladder Resection

If cancer has invaded most of the bladder and excision of the tumor alone is no longer possible, the bladder may have to be removed by open surgery in a procedure called cystectomy. Like radical prostatectomy, this procedure is lengthy and is generally done under general plus epidural anesthesia. The major complications are blood loss and coagulation abnormalities. In this case, coagulation abnormalities occur because the blood being infused lacks certain clotting factors, which can't be preserved as well in stored blood—whether your own or someone else's.

Radical Nephrectomy

Severe infection or cancer may necessitate complete removal of the kidneys. Usually, this operation is performed later in life, which means that patients have numerous coexisting medical conditions.

For kidney removal, patients lie on their side, over a device called a kidney rest that pushes the body upward to expose the flank on the opposite side. Because this positioning is quite uncomfortable, we give general anesthesia unless the patient's medical condition makes it too great a risk. You should also have an epidural, however, for postoperative pain can be considerable.

Because kidney operations can cause wide swings in blood pressure, we place both an arterial line and a central venous pressure catheter. Since the kidney is close to large blood vessels that the surgeon may inadvertently cut—though this is rare—bleeding can be excessive until they're repaired, so preoperative blood donation and autologous blood transfusion are necessary. Frequently, however, patients with diseased kidneys are anemic because their kidneys are not secreting the hormone that stimulates red blood cell production. If this is the case, autologous blood transfusion is not possible, and we must use blood from other donors.

Since kidney operations can take as long as eight hours, we take extra measures to avoid hypothermia: warming the fluids that we administer and covering you with blankets.

- Be sure to ask for an epidural for a radical nephrectomy to control postoperative pain. If epidural anesthesia isn't available, request patient-controlled analgesia. If your blood count is normal, ask for autologous blood transfusion.

Summary: Questions and Points to Remember

- If you're having an extensive bladder tumor removed, request spinal anesthesia—no matter how afraid of it you may be—to reduce the risk of a serious complication.

For radical prostatectomy:

- During the preoperative consultation with your anesthesiologist, ask for an epidural, which can be used for postoperative pain control.
- If you have serious objections to having an epidural for a radical prostatectomy, you can simply refuse—but I don't recommend that you do.
- Ask to donate your blood in advance so it's available for autologous transfusion.

For radical nephrectomy:

- Be sure to ask for an epidural for a radical nephrectomy to control postoperative pain. If epidural anesthesia isn't available, request patient-controlled analgesia.
- If your blood count is normal, ask for autologous blood transfusion.

• • •

CHAPTER 14

Ears, Nose, and Throat

• • •

Many procedures performed on the ears, nose, and throat are quite simple, and are done on an outpatient basis by an otolaryngologist (from the Greek *otos*, for ear, and *larynx*, denoting the upper part of the windpipe). Among these procedures, tonsillectomy and adenoidectomy are covered in chapter 7. Operations to remove cancers of the head and neck, on the other hand, may be long, complex procedures that require a hospital stay.

Middle Ear and Mastoid Surgery

Lost hearing is often the result of a condition that prevents the tiny bones of the middle ear from transmitting sound. The bones may have ossified (hardened), or fluid or debris resulting from chronic infection may obstruct their movement. Microsurgery can restore hearing by releasing the ossification, sucking out fluid, or removing debris.

Often, chronic infection in the mastoid sinuses (air spaces in the bones behind the ears) can affect the ears. When surgery is done to improve hearing, the mastoid sinuses must be resected (partially removed) at the same time, to get rid of the infection completely. This procedure is called mastoidectomy. In someone with a history of chronic infection, it may also be done prophylactically, to prevent hearing loss.

The anesthesiologist's role is particularly demanding in ear procedures. First, since the site of the surgery is so close to the patient's airway, the endotracheal tube must be tightly secured to the patient's face with tape so the surgeon can't dislodge it as he or she works. Second, because the surgeon is working next to the facial nerve, the anesthesiologist must monitor that nerve for signs of injury. Before induction of anesthesia we place a facial nerve stimulator, a monitor that allows us to observe whether administering small amounts of electric current to the facial nerve elicits muscle contractions around the mouth and eyes.

Because the facial twitch must be preserved—so that its absence can serve as an indication that the surgeon has cut or compressed the nerve—we can't completely relax the patient's muscles with muscle relaxants. The anesthesiologist must precisely adjust the dose of muscle relaxant, observing the muscle twitching on the monitor as she or he administers the drug, so that the muscles are relaxed somewhat, but not enough to eliminate the twitch. For this reason some anesthesiologists prefer not to use muscle relaxants at all. However, since the surgery isn't painful, we use only light anesthesia, and without any muscle relaxants it may be difficult to prevent the patient from moving.

I once managed the anesthesia for a friend of mine who had a chronic middle ear infection. During his preoperative consultation I found that he had a history of esophageal varices (a collection of bulging veins in his esophagus, similar to varicose veins), an indication that his liver was damaged. Esophageal varices can occur as a result of liver disease or heavy drinking. Since the varices increased the risk of aspiration of stomach contents, he had to have endotracheal intubation.

Although his history led me to expect that he would require a great deal of anesthesia, it turned out that he required very little, possibly because his liver damage was more extensive than I had thought (see chapter 5, which explains the effects of alcohol on anesthesia). The ear surgeon had asked that I not use large doses of muscle relaxant so we could monitor the patient's facial nerve. But after induction I found that if I used very light anesthesia, he would start moving around on the table; yet when I increased the level of anesthesia, his blood pressure dropped. Since the surgery was being done under a microscope, the surgeon was not too happy about the patient's moving about; but there was nothing I could do. This was one instance where we had no choice but to operate under less than optimal conditions, for the patient's responses wouldn't allow otherwise.

I feared as well that he might experience awareness and either feel pain during the surgery or remember it, so I gave him midazolam to prevent this. After the procedure I went anxiously into the recovery room to see how he was and was quite relieved when he told me cheerfully that he felt fine.

Another possible problem during ear surgery is bleeding, for even tiny amounts of blood will distort the image seen through the microscope. The anesthesiologist therefore uses techniques that prevent bleeding. One is to inject vasoconstrictors (drugs that contract the blood vessels) around the vessels that supply the area being operated on. Since these drugs can cause high blood pressure and abnormal heart rhythms, the anesthesiologist must be alert to correct these conditions should they occur.

Some anesthesiologists also use a technique called deliberate hypotension to prevent bleeding. We reduce the patient's blood pressure by 25 percent of its preoperative level by giving a vasodilator drug (which relaxes the blood vessels), such as nitroprusside, then closely monitoring the blood pressure with an arterial catheter to keep it at a minimal yet safe level.

For ear surgery we avoid using the inhalation anesthetic nitrous oxide, which increases the volume of any air-filled space and would therefore raise pressures in the sinuses and middle ear. This would be particularly dangerous after surgery, for the extra pressure might push the newly fixed bones out of place and rupture the eardrum. Nitrous oxide also makes nausea and vomiting more likely. Since vomiting also raises pressure inside the head, it's important to prevent these patients from feeling nauseated. Postoperative nausea and vomiting are common anyway after ear surgery, so you should be given intravenous antiemetics (drugs that prevent it) at least an hour before the end of the procedure.

- Ask your anesthesiologist to administer antiemetic drugs during your surgery.

Since patients don't experience severe pain after this surgery, low-dose intramuscular narcotics are often adequate for pain relief.

- If the narcotics you're given don't completely relieve your postsurgical pain, ask for a higher dose.

Surgery on the Vocal Cords

People who develop hoarseness or a chronic cough frequently need surgery to remove polyps (growths on mucous membranes) from their vocal cords.

Diagnosis

The surgeon performs a diagnostic laryngoscopy (using an endoscope designed to look directly at the larynx, or voicebox), searching either for polyps or for a nerve paralysis that would prevent one vocal cord from moving. Laryngoscopy is done under general anesthesia, using only large doses of induction drugs such as propofol or thiopental, since the procedure is quite short. The anesthesiologist also sprays the vocal cords with a local anesthetic and administers local anesthetics intravenously to decrease the chance that the patient will cough when the surgeon inserts the laryngoscope. Some surgeons also apply cocaine as a local anesthetic; when this is done, the anesthesiologist must be prepared to treat hypertension.

If you have preexisting hypertension, whether treated or untreated, you might need some other form of anesthesia for laryngoscopy, such as local blocks of the nerves that innervate the throat. (See chapter 2 for a description of how inhalation anesthetics affect people with high blood pressure and chapter 5 for the effects of cocaine.)

- During the preoperative consultation, be sure to tell the anesthesiologist if you have high blood pressure so that he or she will not use drugs that increase hypertension.

Anesthesia during Surgery

Surgery on the vocal cords is done with lasers. The complications that may occur during these procedures require specific precautions and advance preparation, making a preoperative visit to the anesthesiologist mandatory. During this consultation the anesthesiologist evaluates your degree of hoarseness and/or the severity of your cough. If either is considerable, you will need an additional examination under direct vision (laryngoscopy) so the anesthesiologist can assess whether the airway will be difficult to control. Also, since the laser can cause fires in the trachea, we use special endotracheal tubes made of noncombustible materials.

Endotracheal intubation is necessary because the surgery is done within the airway itself. We give general anesthesia, since sedation and analgesia, even combined with local blocks, would not prevent the surgery from stimulating laryngospasm (contraction of the throat muscles), and the patient would be unable to breathe. For the general, we avoid nitrous oxide and use only a minimal amount of oxygen, since both these gases will worsen any fires started by the laser.

We also use the smallest-diameter tube possible that will still allow gas exchange in the lungs, since the surgeon is working in the same opening at the top of the trachea that the tube passes through. Because of these tight conditions, there's a chance that the surgeon might inadvertently pull the tube out an inch or two, so it's no longer reaching the lung, or flatten it against the wall of the trachea, so that air can't get through. The anesthesiologist—who backs away from the operating table while the surgeon works—must listen vigilantly to the patient's breath sounds and closely watch the end-tidal carbon dioxide monitor showing the amount of carbon dioxide leaving the lungs at the end of each breath, so that if the tube is dislodged she or he can instantly ask the surgeon to replace it.

Recovery

The good news is that you won't have pain after vocal cord surgery—not even much of a sore throat. The problem we do need to avoid, however, is coughing spasms. Your anesthesiologist should ask the surgeon to place local anesthetic blocks around your vocal cords once surgery is complete to prevent irritation that would lead to coughing. The anesthesiologist can also administer local anesthetics intravenously; these work systemically to decrease the cough reflex. These IV anesthetics can be repeated at intervals if coughing recurs. Finally, you can self-administer local anesthetics from a nebulizer.

Nasal Surgery

Surgery on the nose and sinuses comprises a large part of the otolaryngologist's practice. Common procedures include reconstruction of the nasal septum (the structure that separates the two nasal cavities), submucous resection (removal of swollen and inflamed mucous membranes to correct breathing problems), removal of nasal polyps, and various procedures on the nasal sinuses to eliminate chronic infection.

Nasal surgery may be an open procedure but is also—depending on the surgeon's skills—often performed endoscopically, with the endoscope passed up through the nose. During endoscopic procedures, large doses of local anesthetics mixed with vasoconstrictors are usually injected into the operative site to decrease bleeding and thereby increase visibility through the scope.

Anesthesia is similar for all these procedures. The choice is between general anesthesia and local anesthesia with sedation; it should be made in consultation with the surgeon, for it depends on how extensive the procedure will be. If the procedure is simple, we generally do it under sedation and analgesia, using propofol and short-acting intravenous narcotics. In addition, the surgeon injects local anesthetics directly into the area being operated on; the drugs most commonly used are cocaine and lidocaine with epinephrine, which produce both analgesia and vasoconstriction. For extensive procedures, you should request general anesthesia. In fact, since bone, cartilage, and mucous membrane are being resected, these procedures are extremely painful, so most people prefer general anesthesia. We also give an antiemetic to help prevent nausea and vomiting.

Nasal surgery presents several challenges to the anesthesiologist. First, too much local anesthetic injected into the operative site and absorbed into the body can cause systemic toxicity, resulting in seizures and cardiac dysrhythmias (abnormal heart rhythms). Second, the vasoconstrictors used can lead to hypertension and increase the risk of cardiac dysrhythmias. Third, some inhalation anesthetics used for general anesthesia sensitize the heart to the effects of vasoconstrictors and increase the possibility of severe dysrhythmias. Nevertheless we use these drugs because they make it easier to control increases in blood pressure caused by the vasoconstrictors. Fourth, since the surgery manipulates areas adjacent to the breathing tube, the tube can be easily dislodged, so the anesthesiologist must constantly listen to breath sounds and observe the end-tidal carbon dioxide monitor. And finally, since the nasal area has a rich supply of blood vessels, blood loss can be significant.

- Be sure to tell your anesthesiologist if you have a history of hypertension or cardiac dysrhythmias, for in these cases the choice and dose of vasoconstrictor to be used must be made extremely carefully.

After surgery, all your nasal passages will be packed to decrease the chance of bleeding, so the anesthesiologist must take great care to ensure that you can breathe. You'll have to breathe through your mouth, which often makes nausea and vomiting more likely. For this reason you should receive liberal doses of antiemetics.

- If you become nauseous easily, ask the anesthesiologist to give you an antiemetic before you leave the operating room.

Complex procedures performed under general anesthesia may require that you stay in the hospital as long as twenty-three hours (under twenty-four hours you're still considered ambulatory). In such a case you'll need postoperative pain control. Immediate postoperative pain can be decreased by an injection of local anesthetic into the operative site just before the end of surgery. Within four hours after you leave the operating room, however, you should receive injected narcotics to relieve pain for the first twenty-four hours after surgery. You can then go home with oral narcotics to control any remaining pain. Bear in mind that narcotics may increase the nausea associated with these procedures, so you may do better with nonsteroidal anti-inflammatory drugs as your pain subsides.

- If narcotics make you nauseous and NSAIDs don't, ask for the nonsteroidals instead.

Surgery for Cancers of the Head and Neck

Complex procedures to resect carcinoma of the head and neck are generally performed for people who already have complicated medical histories. Cancer of the tongue or of the back of the pharynx (throat), for example, usually occurs after years of smoking and drinking. Consequently, the patients may also have chronic lung disease and cirrhosis of the liver, and these conditions must be controlled as well as possible before anesthesia and surgery.

To evaluate and stage (determine the phase of progression of) cancers of the head and neck, you may have a procedure called a panendoscopy, in which the scope is passed through the larynx into the trachea, then down the esophagus. It's a simple procedure that's usually done under sedation and analgesia but may be performed under general anesthesia.

- If you feel having panendoscopy under sedation and analgesia would be too uncomfortable, you can request general anesthesia.

Preoperative Consultation

If you have complex medical problems, you should see your anesthesiologist at least one week, and preferably two weeks, before surgery. He or she will examine your lungs and measure your arterial blood gas to see whether further pulmonary function testing (which measures how well your lungs work) is needed. Patients who have been heavy drinkers also need a liver function test to determine how much liver function is present. Liver testing is particularly important because some anesthetic drugs are metabolized by the liver, and if the liver can't perform this function adequately during a long procedure, the drugs will build up in the body, and the patient will take longer to wake up after surgery.

- If you have chronic lung disease or cirrhosis of the liver, see your internist just before you see your anesthesiologist. Bring the anesthesiologist all the information about your condition.
- Continue taking all your regular medications during the two weeks before surgery.

The anesthesiologist also assesses the drugs you're taking, paying particular attention to the use of bronchodilators (drugs that make breathing easier by opening the airways), since these drugs must be available during induction of anesthesia in case bronchospasm (contraction of the airways) occurs. A cough that produces yellow sputum indicates that chest infection is present, and you will need to take antibiotics before surgery.

- During the two-week period before surgery, stop smoking if you possibly can.

The tumor itself often causes problems that complicate anesthetic management, and the anesthesiologist will look for these too during the preoperative visit. Sometimes the tumor interferes with eating, and the anesthesiologist must note any resulting malnutrition, anemia, or dehydration. We assess whether your fluid volume is too low by looking directly for dehydrated mucous membranes (such as a dry tongue). We also do blood tests to look for abnormalities in your electrolytes (substances essential for conduction of nerve impulses, which must be present in precise proportions in the serum) and to measure serum proteins, which indicate the degree of malnutrition. Low protein levels would prevent or increase the action of some anesthetic drugs. To correct imbalances, before surgery we give intravenous fluids containing needed electrolytes.

The tumor may also compress the airway, as may enlarged lymph nodes associated with the cancer. For this reason, the anesthesiologist needs to directly visualize the opening of the trachea with a laryngoscope before inducing anesthesia, to make sure nothing is blocking it. A tumor may also compress the airway below the larynx, preventing the endotracheal tube from passing into the lungs. If the anesthesiologist's examination indicates that she or he may be unable to intubate you, you may have the choice to undergo an attempted intubation while awake, after appropriate nerve blocks with local anesthesia and inhaled xylocaine. If this is not possible, you will need a tracheostomy, in which the surgeon, after injecting local anesthetics, inserts the breathing tube through an incision made in the wall of the trachea before general anesthesia is induced. If awake intubation is possible, I recommend it; it's less anxiety-provoking, and it doesn't leave you with a scar.

Anesthesia during Surgery

The complexity and duration of these procedures make general anesthesia mandatory. We choose inhalation anesthetics, such as isoflurane, and muscle relaxants that are not metabolized by the liver. We place an arterial line to monitor changes in blood pressure due to excessive blood loss, and a central venous pressure catheter, which is inserted into a major vein to monitor the volume and pressure of blood returning to the heart. This is necessary since in people with chronic lung disease, right heart failure may occur. Last, because the operation is so long, we place a Foley catheter; otherwise, urine would build up and the distended bladder could cause hypotension and rapid heartbeat, among other problems.

To prevent a drop in body temperature, which is likely during long procedures, we use a warming blanket, a device that resembles an air mattress through which warm air is blown. In addition, we warm the blood and other fluids we administer by running the tubing that carries them through a machine called a fluid warmer.

Relatives of patients having this type of surgery should be aware that the procedure can take twelve to fourteen hours. The patient will then probably stay overnight in the recovery room.

- Don't worry if your family member is in the operating room for many hours.
- Try to remain with the patient during the postoperative period, watching to be sure the tracheostomy tube remains in place.

Recovery

If you've had a tracheostomy, the staff members who transport you out of the operating room must be extra careful to avoid inadvertent removal of the tube from your throat. When the tube is pulled out of a fresh tracheostomy, the opening closes up and we can't easily see where it is to replace the tube.

Since during the operation large amounts of fluid are absorbed into the tissues around the operative site, postoperatively the anesthesiologist must pay careful attention to managing your fluid volume and electrolyte balance by appropriate monitoring while you're in the intensive care unit. You'll need pain control with narcotics, administered either by PCA or by intramuscular injections. You can expect to remain in the ICU for two to three days before being transferred to a regular unit.

Summary: Questions and Points to Remember

For ear surgery:

- Ask your anesthesiologist to administer antiemetic drugs during your surgery.

- If the narcotics you're given don't completely relieve your postsurgical pain, ask for a higher dose.

For vocal cord surgery:

- During the preoperative consultation, be sure to tell the anesthesiologist if you have high blood pressure so that he or she will not use drugs that increase hypertension.

For nasal surgery:

- Be sure to tell your anesthesiologist if you have a history of hypertension or cardiac dysrhythmias, for in these cases the choice and dose of vasoconstrictor to be used must be made extremely carefully.
- If you become nauseous easily, ask the anesthesiologist to give you an antiemetic before you leave the operating room.
- If narcotics make you nauseous and NSAIDs don't, ask for the nonsteroidals instead.

For surgery for head or neck cancers:

- If you feel having panendoscopy under sedation and analgesia would be too uncomfortable, you can request general anesthesia.
- If you have chronic lung disease or cirrhosis of the liver, see your internist just before you see your anesthesiologist. Bring the anesthesiologist all the information about your condition.
- Continue taking all your regular medications during the two weeks before surgery.
- During the two-week period before surgery, stop smoking if you possibly can.
- Don't worry if your family member is in the operating room for many hours.
- Try to remain with the patient during the postoperative period, watching to be sure the tracheostomy tube remains in place.

• • •

Other Types
of Ambulatory Surgery

• • •

Let me walk you through a typical ambulatory surgery experience with fifty-four-year-old Arlene. She went to her primary care physician to have the burning, itching pain that occurred when she sat too long at her desk checked out and learned she had hemorrhoids that required surgery. The doctor referred Arlene to a surgeon at our hospital's ambulatory surgery center, whom she saw at his private office (she could also have seen him during his office hours at the hospital). After he evaluated her and discussed the plan for surgery, she was scheduled to see the anesthesiologist at the hospital within two weeks prior to surgery for a complete evaluation of her medical condition and to develop an anesthetic plan.

For many patients, this preadmission visit means spending a marathon day at the hospital, visiting not just the anesthesiologist but the laboratory for blood tests and an electrocardiogram, as well as the radiology department for other tests the surgeon has ordered. Patients with no serious disease and who are not having complex surgery usually don't need any testing, except that women of childbearing age may have a pregnancy test. But those with significant medical problems will need, for example, an electrocardiogram to evaluate heart function, or maybe a chest x-ray if they have a cough. If the anesthesiologist wants any additional tests, she or he will order these to be done while the patient is at the hospital. We try get all the tests completed on a single day; some centers have evening or Saturday hours to make this possible.

If you do have tests, when the results come back from the lab, a nurse checks them, and if they aren't normal, the surgeon or anesthesiologist determines whether you need treatment by your primary care doctor to correct the abnormalities. The two-week period usually allows enough time to do this without delaying the surgery.

Some hospitals will instead first give you a questionnaire developed by the anesthesia department that covers your medical and anesthesia history, medications used, and allergies. It's important to fill it out accurately, for your answers are likely to determine what type of anesthesia you will receive and whether or not you see an anesthesia provider before your surgery. The more complex your preexisting medical conditions and the procedure you'll be having, the more likely it is that you'll see an anesthesiologist during this preadmission visit. At other centers, if you don't need any lab tests, a nurse calls you and takes your history over the phone, then decides whether you need to come in to meet with the anesthesiologist; the nurse also gives you instructions for the day of surgery. Remember, if you want to see an anesthesiologist, you can always request this, even if you're not having lab tests.

Arlene, being relatively healthy and not of childbearing age, needed no tests, so from the anesthesiologist she went to see a nurse in the ambulatory surgery unit, who told her when to arrive at the hospital on the day of her surgery and instructed her not to eat or drink anything for eight hours before that time. Last, the nurse explained that Arlene would need someone to take her home afterward.

On the day of surgery, Arlene arrived at the scheduled time and was admitted to the ambulatory surgery unit. Here a nurse checked her vital signs and completed a checklist to make sure her chart contained the notes left by the surgeon, anesthesiologist, and other staff members who had seen her, as well as her signed consent form. If Arlene had had lab tests, the nurse would also have checked to be sure the latest results were in the chart and were within normal limits.

Next, Arlene was brought to a holding area, where another nurse started an intravenous line in the back of Arlene's hand. Here she met the anesthesiologist who would be administering her anesthesia. He explained what he would be doing, then escorted her as she walked, trailing her IV pole, to the operating room. Since Arlene was quite calm, she received no sedatives. If she'd been very anxious, the anesthesiologist would have given her a sedative through the IV line and taken her to the operating room on a stretcher.

Arlene's daughter, Carla, who had brought her to the hospital, stayed with her up to the moment when she left for the operating room. Although the nurse told Carla she could leave and return in an hour and a half to pick her mother up, Carla decided to stay in the adjacent family waiting room.

Meanwhile Arlene, in the operating room, was connected to the routine monitors: a blood pressure cuff on her arm, a temperature probe in her armpit, and a pulse oximeter on her finger. The anesthesiologist gave her intravenous midazolam to sedate her and, briefly, fentanyl to provide analgesia while he administered local anesthesia for the surgery. She was then turned on her side, so he could give her a spinal.

After making sure the anesthesia was adequate, the surgeon began to operate. Before long the surgery was complete; the entire procedure, including administration of anesthesia, had taken thirty minutes. Arlene was now placed on a stretcher and taken to the ambulatory surgery recovery room. Unlike the recovery room in regular surgical units, here families are encouraged to stay with the patient and to offer juice and toast, since the ability to eat and not become nauseous shows that the patient is ready for discharge.

After about forty-five minutes in the recovery room, Arlene was asked to walk to the ambulatory surgery nursing unit, where a nurse observed her to be sure she was ready to leave. Arlene and Carla then met with the nurse, who described potential problems to watch for: weakness in the legs, which could indicate that the anesthesia was still effective, and bleeding from the operative site. The nurse told Arlene that if she had excessive bleeding or had trouble urinating she should return immediately to the hospital or contact the surgeon directly, and gave her the numbers to call. Last, the nurse gave her prescriptions that the surgeon had written for pain relievers. In some hospitals and freestanding ambulatory surgery centers, these prescriptions can be filled in the pharmacy before the patient leaves.

I want to emphasize that Carla's presence during this review of the discharge instructions was essential, for it was her knowledge of what problems to look for and how to react to them that would ensure her mother's continued safe recovery at home.

- If you're having ambulatory surgery, the friend or family member who brings you home should sit in on your final conference with the nurse before discharge.

Ensuring Quality of Care

Ambulatory surgery has become increasingly popular since the early 1980s—made possible, as I noted in chapter 2, by the development of anesthetic drugs that leave the body rapidly, have fewer side effects, such as nausea and vomiting, and have few if any residual effects, such as fatigue or sleepiness. In the beginning, mostly minor procedures, such as breast biopsies, were performed on patients who had no preexisting medical problems. By the 1990s, however, even people with complicated diseases, who needed complex procedures, were having surgery as outpatients. These procedures were being performed in ambulatory surgery units in major medical centers and in small community hospitals, as well as in freestanding facilities specializing in ambulatory surgery. At present, at least 65 percent of all surgical procedures in the United States are performed in outpatient facilities.

Complications after ambulatory surgery are extremely rare, thanks to measures that safeguard quality of care. During the 1990s, standards of care governing hospital facilities and the qualifications of the personnel who worked there were developed by representatives of anesthesia and hospital organizations and implemented by the Joint Commission for Accreditation of Hospital Organizations, an industry group. Ambulatory surgery units in major academic medical centers and in community hospitals are inspected periodically by the JCAHO to ensure that they adhere to these standards. If you have surgery in a facility approved by the JCAHO, you can be assured that you'll receive a high level of care.

Freestanding ambulatory surgery centers must be licensed and are frequently accredited by the American Association for Ambulatory Health Care, whose standards are similar to those of the JCAHO. Some state health departments also inspect and accredit these facilities. These centers may provide high-quality care, but since they don't have the same resources as hospitals, they may not be appropriate for complex surgical procedures on patients with complicated medical problems. People with severe asthma, sickle cell anemia, uncontrolled high blood pressure, coronary artery disease, and hemophilia or another blood-clotting disorder, as well as extremely obese people, should not have ambulatory surgery and are best observed overnight in a hospital.

The anesthetics used for most of these patients are short-acting intravenous drugs and the newer inhalants, which are expired from the body within minutes after being discontinued. New short-acting muscle relaxants are also available, should muscle relaxation be necessary. The following sections describe the anesthetic considerations specific to all the most common ambulatory procedures not covered by previous chapters.

General Surgery

Hernias. Hernias occur around the umbilicus (navel), in the abdomen, or in the groin. They are usually repaired by a general surgeon, under regional or general anesthesia. Both types of anesthesia last about the same length of time, so the choice does not affect the time of your discharge. Regional anesthesia does have two advantages. First, you can be awake during the procedure, which your surgeon sometimes prefers. He or she may, for example, want to ask you to force a cough during the procedure in order to check the integrity of the repair. Second, there is generally less postoperative nausea and vomiting.

Small hernias around or close to the umbilicus can be repaired using only IV sedation, with local anesthesia applied to the wound. Larger umbilical hernias, however, require regional anesthesia that affects nerves and muscles at a higher level in the body and might result in an uncomfortable feeling of not being able to breathe deeply. In addition, you might experience cramps during the surgery due to stimulation of the intestines on the side of the hernia. Thus you might consider requesting general anesthesia for these hernias.

With inguinal hernias, these problems don't occur, so for those, regional anesthesia—either a spinal or an epidural—is best. Most often we do a spinal because it's easier to administer, but we can give an epidural. We can also include a narcotic in the spinal or epidural that adds to postsurgical pain relief. And in addition, the surgeon can inject a long-acting local anesthetic into the operative area to control pain for up to four hours after surgery. You'll be most comfortable if you have both the narcotic and the long-acting local together.

- Ask your surgeon to give you a long-acting local anesthetic in addition to the spinal or epidural you receive.
- If you've had a spinal or epidural, tell the nurse if your legs are weak or you have difficulty walking or urinating.

If you do, you should not be discharged; it usually takes about two hours from the time you get the spinal or epidural until these symptoms wear off.

Gallbladder Removal. Gallbladders are now removed laparoscopically, which is to say through a tube inserted into a small incision made in the abdomen. During the surgery, carbon dioxide is injected into the abdomen; the gas expands the abdominal wall away from the gallbladder, making this organ easier to see. The gas builds up in the blood and must be exhaled. For this reason general anesthesia is necessary so that the anesthesiologist can eliminate the gas adequately by controlling the patient's breathing.

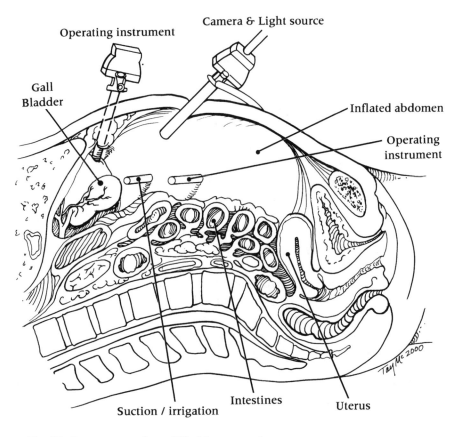

Fig. 17. *Laparoscopy for gallbladder removal.*

Since the incision is small, postoperative pain after gallbladder excision is minimal. However, you can expect to stay in the ambulatory surgery facility for ten to twenty-three hours, since this procedure often results in postoperative nausea and vomiting.

- In scheduling your surgery, anticipate an extended stay in the recovery facility and time it to be most comfortable and convenient.

If your surgery takes place early in the morning, you can go home the same night; while if you have surgery later in the day, you may wind up staying in the hospital overnight.

Intestinal Adhesions. Adhesions are fibrous bands of scar tissue that sometimes develop in the intestines and adjacent structures after abdominal or gynecological surgery. They can cause abdominal pain and even obstruction of bowel movements. (When the bowels are already ob-structed—a serious problem—surgery to remove adhesions must be done as an emergency procedure and therefore isn't ambulatory, since you're admitted to the hospital emergency room.) The surgeon searches for and resects (removes) the adhesions through a laparoscope.

This procedure can be performed under regional anesthesia. However, since a gas is injected into the abdomen to improve visualization of the adhesions, if you are unable to breathe rapidly to eliminate it, you may need general anesthesia. Unlike gallbladder removal, where the anesthetic is likely to impair breathing because it is administered higher up in the body, removal of adhesions is done at a lower level, so you might be able to breathe rapidly and have a regional. But you might consider having a general anyway, to avoid cramping caused by the distention of the entire abdomen by the gas.

Postoperative pain is minimal after this procedure, but you can expect abdominal cramps, nausea, and vomiting. We give you narcotics for the cramps and antiemetics to control nausea and vomiting.

Procedures on the Eye

Procedures performed on the eye pose a particular challenge for the an-esthesiologist. There is a reflex between the eye and the heart, such that when the eye is stimulated, the heart rate slows significantly. During any eye procedure, therefore, the anesthesiologist must watch for cardiac prob-lems and be prepared to treat them by administering appropriate drugs to speed the heart up.

- If you are having eye surgery, be sure an anesthesiologist is readily available.

The local anesthetics used during eye surgery should provide long-lasting postoperative pain relief. If you have significant pain after surgery, contact your surgeon immediately.

Cataract Removal. People who need cataracts removed are generally older and likely to have complicated medical problems. They can usually be treated as outpatients, but they must see an anesthesiologist preopera-tively to ensure that their preexisting diseases are properly managed and that the anesthetics chosen are tailored for their medical conditions. Patients are usually asked to come to the hospital about two hours in advance of surgery, since drops must be placed in their eyes to dilate the pupils.

Since cataract removal may require a local anesthetic block placed right into the eye, we administer intravenous anesthetics that induce brief loss of consciousness just before the ophthalmologist or anesthesiologist injects the block. Giving general anesthesia, even this briefly, to an older patient with complex conditions requires close monitoring by the anesthesiologist. Once the local anesthetic has taken effect, the patient regains consciousness and remains awake for the rest of the procedure, while sedation is continued at a reduced level. We cover you with warm sheets to keep you comfortable. Since it's important that you remain still during the surgery, let us know if there's a particular position that's more comfortable for you. We can usually prop a pillow under your back or legs.

Cataract patients who are elderly and sick need someone to accompany them to and from the hospital. And since one eye will be bandaged after the operation, I strongly recommend that all such patients have someone stay overnight with them after surgery.

Retinal Detachment. Retinal detachment, a condition in which the light-sensitive inner layer of the eyeball separates from the underlying nutrient layer, can occur at any age; when it does, it requires immediate attention. Some people need emergency surgery to prevent injury to the retina and resulting loss of vision. Since these patients are likely to have full stomachs, we can't give them sedation and analgesia because of the risk of vomiting and aspiration of stomach contents into the lungs. When it's not an emergency, the repair can be done as a scheduled procedure under intravenous sedation and retrobulbar block (placed behind the eye), or, if necessary, under general anesthesia. Younger, healthy people may be able to have light sedation and analgesia that calms them but doesn't cause loss of consciousness. The local anesthetic block provides postoperative pain control.

Glaucoma. Glaucoma is a condition of increased pressure within the eye, resulting in diminished blood flow to the optic nerve, which in turn causes loss of vision. Various procedures to reduce this pressure are commonly done as ambulatory surgery. Sometimes a laser is used to open up the channels by which liquid flows in and out of the chambers of the eye. If this treatment fails, a more invasive drainage procedure called trabeculectomy is necessary to unblock the trabecular meshwork, a delicate structure through which liquid flows. The surgeon drills a hole in the trabecular meshwork to allow drainage from the chambers of the eye, thus decreasing the pressure. This procedure is generally done under IV sedation and local anesthesia.

Dental Rehabilitation and Extraction

Often people need tooth extractions and other types of dental procedures (rehabilitation) that are more extensive than dentists can perform in an office and require more analgesia than nitrous oxide (the dentist's standard inhalant anesthetic) can provide. These procedures are performed in an ambulatory surgery setting under general anesthesia. Patients are treated like any other patient having general anesthesia, with a preoperative visit for a complete evaluation and treatment of any preexisting conditions before the date of surgery.

General anesthesia is administered through an endotracheal tube that is usually inserted through the nostril so that the oral surgeon can work in the mouth without risk of dislodging it. After the surgery, you can expect nausea and vomiting in reaction to blood in your mouth or stomach. To minimize this we usually suction out the stomach before the surgery is over and give an antiemetic.

Another group for whom the ambulatory surgery setting is appropriate is the mentally challenged, who, even more than other patients, need a thorough preoperative consultation because of the possibility that existing abnormalities could lead to problems during anesthesia. For example, before having a dental extraction or rehabilitation, a person with Down's syndrome must be thoroughly evaluated for other congenital anomalies, such as heart or facial deformities; the latter may make it difficult to manage the airway. When the patient has a history of seizures, the condition should be well controlled, and the patient must continue taking medication through the day of the surgery.

Often, mentally challenged patients need to be heavily sedated prior to dental procedures because of their inability to cooperate. We do this by administering midazolam via the mouth or rectum, as described in chapter 2. Once sedated, the patient can be taken to the operating room and given general anesthesia. Postoperatively, a mentally challenged patient must be completely awake before the tube is removed, since it would be difficult to reinsert should breathing problems occur.

Plastic Surgery

The popularity of plastic surgery increased rapidly during the 1990s. Common procedures now include facelifts (rhytidectomy), nose jobs (rhinoplasty), eyelid tucks (blepharoplasty), and liposuction. These operations are performed both in ambulatory surgery centers and in physicians' offices.

As I noted in chapter 2, the practice of office-based surgery is so new that standards of care for this setting are just now being developed. It's therefore crucial to be sure that resuscitation equipment and properly trained staff are present for any procedure you undergo in a doctor's office. Please read the cautions in the section "Office-Based Anesthesia and Surgery" in chapter 2 and ask the questions listed there.

Facelifts. An anesthesiologist should be present during a facelift, for a number of reasons. First, deep sedation is required, since any movement by the patient would have a disastrous effect on the results. (Sometimes general anesthesia is used, but the breathing tube extending from the mouth may pull on one side of the face, affecting the results.) Second, if the patient moves, there is a risk of damage to the facial nerve that could cause facial paralysis. Third, since bleeding during a facelift may be excessive, fluid volume must be closely monitored so that you can be resuscitated, if necessary.

After this operation, you may have significant pain, which is controlled by pain medications prescribed by the surgeon. Since a facelift can take six to eight hours, during all of which you are heavily sedated, you may feel drowsy for some time afterward. It's therefore mandatory that someone accompany you home and stay the night with you. If you are excessively sleepy, you should take pain medication sparingly or not at all.

People with serious medical conditions should have facelifts done in hospital-based ambulatory surgery centers, not in a doctor's office.

Nose Jobs. People have nose jobs not only for cosmetic reasons but also because of breathing problems. Rhinoplasty is quite painful, since bone is being broken, so you will need deep sedation administered by the anesthesiologist plus an injection of local anesthetic by the surgeon. Since the surgeon also uses a vasoconstrictor, such as adrenaline, to minimize bleeding, the anesthesiologist must pay careful attention to possible increases in blood pressure. (See chapter 5 for a description of the effects of cocaine on blood pressure.)

- If you have a history of high blood pressure, be sure all the people involved in the procedure know about it. The anesthesiologist must be prepared for a sudden rise in blood pressure so she or he can treat it immediately.

If you prefer, you can have general anesthesia for a nose job. Again, however, because the breathing tube is so close to the operative site, this will make it harder for the surgeon to perform the procedure. For cosmetic reasons, then, it's probably best to have sedation and analgesia.

Eye Tucks. Since eyelid procedures are less painful than the other cosmetic procedures described here, they're generally performed under light sedation combined with local anesthesia.

Liposuction. Excess fat can be removed from almost any part of the body by liposuction. Since this procedure is quite painful, you need general anesthesia. In addition to pain, liposuction may cause a significant loss of body fluids, which can result in acidosis, an excess accumulation of acid in the body that may lead to heart failure. Because of this danger, an anesthesiologist should be present during the procedure to prevent acidosis by administering fluids.

If you are having liposuction on several parts of your body, it's probably best to do it in stages, since there have been reports that people who had extensive liposuction in a single procedure have gone home and died from the effects of acidosis. Other reports indicate that some plastic surgeons may use large amounts of lidocaine during liposuction. These high doses can be toxic and cause cardiac arrest. Deaths after liposuction from all causes have been reported as 1 in 5,000. This is not a benign procedure.

- If you're having liposuction, have it done in stages and request that an anesthesiologist be present for sedation and analgesia. Check to make sure that your surgeon is qualified to perform this procedure and whether there are any complications on his or her record. You can call your state health department to see if this information is available where you live.

Colonoscopy

Colonoscopy, a diagnostic procedure performed to check for colon cancer, is now recommended every two to four years for people over fifty. The entire colon is visually examined with a colonoscope, a flexible tube with a light at the end. In order to visualize the colon well, the gastroenterologist distends it by injecting gas through a side port in the scope. Insertion of the tube and distention of the bowel are uncomfortable, requiring intravenous midazolam for sedation and narcotics to control pain.

Whether or not you need an anesthesiologist present depends on your medical condition. If you have significant medical problems, an anesthesiologist should be there. If you don't, at least one other staff person trained in resuscitation should be present, since the person performing the colonoscopy will not be able to monitor your condition and resuscitate you if necessary. In either case, the facility should have available the necessary resuscitation equipment and drugs.

After a colonoscopy you may experience severe cramping—usually resulting from the insufflated gas—that simulates gas pains. Most often you can pass this gas, making sedation and painkillers unnecessary.

- Don't hesitate to pass gas in the recovery area. If you don't, you will only become more uncomfortable and your return home will be delayed.
- Should the pain last longer than six hours, you should return to the physician who performed the colonoscopy, since this pain may signal a perforation of the bowel.

Summary: Questions and Points to Remember

- If you're having ambulatory surgery, the friend or family member who brings you home should sit in on your final conference with the nurse before discharge.
- In scheduling gallbladder removal, anticipate an extended stay in the recovery facility and time it to be most comfortable and convenient.
- If you are having eye surgery, be sure an anesthesiologist is readily available.

For hernia procedures:

- Ask your surgeon to give you a long-acting local anesthetic in addition to the spinal or epidural you receive. If you've had a spinal or epidural, tell the nurse if your legs are weak or you have difficulty walking or urinating.

For plastic surgery:

- If you are having a nose job and have a history of high blood pressure, be sure all the people involved in the procedure know about it. If you're having liposuction, have it done in stages and request that an anesthesiologist be present for sedation and analgesia. Check to make sure that your surgeon is qualified to perform liposuction and whether there are any complications on his or her record.

After colonoscopy:

- Don't hesitate to pass gas in the recovery area. Should the pain last longer than six hours, you should return to the physician who performed the colonoscopy, since this pain may signal a perforation of the bowel.

CHAPTER 16

• • •

Chronic Pain Management

• • •

One Christmas a few years ago, I visited my nephew and his family. After dinner we were sitting around the tree, when suddenly Santa Claus rang the doorbell. In came a large, jolly man in a Santa suit, a bag of presents slung over his back. He distributed the gifts to the children, then stayed for coffee and cookies.

As we talked, I discovered that this was his first day out of bed in a long time. For years Richard had been felled by severe low back pain. Three operations by a neurosurgeon had failed to relieve it; so had oral narcotics and narcotic patches in ever larger doses. Not only did his pain persist, but the drugs left him dopey and nauseous. No physician could discover the cause of the pain, and with his mind constantly fuzzy, he found himself, at forty-four, unable to work (he was a police officer).

Luckily, a friend recommended him to my nephew, an anesthesiologist who specializes in pain management. After a work-up that ruled out a slipped disk, my nephew implanted an infusion pump under Richard's skin. From the pump, an intrathecal catheter (one inserted into the sheath surrounding the spinal cord) was tunneled under the skin and into the spinal canal at the upper part of his low back. A continuous infusion of the narcotic fentanyl into the spinal canal completely relieved Richard's pain, without any side effects. He was ready to go back to work. His appearance as Santa was his way of expressing his jubilation and his gratitude to my nephew.

Advances in Treating Chronic Pain

The ability to relieve certain types of chronic pain with nerve blocks and implantable devices like Richard's pump constitutes one of the most significant advances in anesthesiology today. New technology allows us to place catheters in precise locations either inside or just outside the spinal canal, and to place electronic stimulators on particular areas of the spine.

Most of these procedures are performed under fluoroscopy (x-ray guidance), which enables the pain specialist to position the device in precisely the right location both to relieve the pain and to avoid serious complications, such as paraplegia (paralysis of the legs). Physicians who perform these procedures must work closely with specialized companies that provide up-to-the-minute equipment and instruction in using it.

A Shift in Attitudes

These technological advances have accompanied a welcome shift in attitudes toward pain on the part of both doctors and patients. As I noted in the introduction, physicians have traditionally been unresponsive to patients' pain. Even today, medical schools and residency programs typically offer little if any instruction in pain management. Only recently, for example, has the medical school where I teach added pain management to its curriculum. As a result of this lack of education, many physicians remain reluctant to prescribe powerful painkillers. One reason is that they fear their patients will turn into addicts. Another is fear that if they use narcotics too aggressively, they will face scrutiny by state and federal authorities, which sometimes take action against doctors and pharmacists for what is considered overuse of these drugs. Even doctors who are more willing to prescribe narcotics for people with terminal illnesses may refuse to give them to people with chronic pain—especially those receiving workers' compensation payments, who are suspected of malingering.

For their part, many patients are equally afraid of becoming addicts if they take narcotics. Or, clinging to the old belief that bearing pain stoically is a sign of moral virtue, they don't even ask their doctors for adequate pain relief. As a result of this complex of attitudes, many people continue to suffer chronic pain that could be relieved.

Fortunately, this situation is beginning to change. In 1999 the Oregon Board of Medical Examiners disciplined a physician for inadequately treating his patients' pain. According to the *New York Times*, advocates of improved pain treatment saw this case as an indication not only of a shift in the medical community's attitudes but also of a major change in the public's feelings about how pain should be managed. Some medical schools are introducing new curricula for teaching not just pain management but also palliative medicine, a field that covers both pain control and the psychological suffering of dying patients and their families. The Joint Commission for Accreditation of Hospital Organizations has mandated that, starting in the year 2000, hospitals must address all patients' pain; this is not a choice, but a requirement. And the Agency for Health Care Policy and Research, part of the federal Department of Health and Human Services, issued clinical practice guidelines saying that hospitals should treat acute and chronic pain aggressively with powerful narcotics. In 1999 the AHCPR was renamed Agency for Healthcare Research and Quality. You can find the guidelines at its website: http://www.ahcpr.gov/clinic/medtep/acute.htm. Although these guidelines are voluntary, you can use them to support requests for treatment of your own pain.

- In discussing your pain with your doctor, refer to these guidelines as an appropriate standard for your care.

Another component of the changes underway is the creation of credentialing programs for pain specialists. Since 1990 formal training programs have been developed to teach anesthesiologists and other physicians how to manage complex pain conditions. Official credentialing boards award certificates to physicians who meet their requirements. In 1996 the American Board of Anesthesiology initiated a requirement for an additional year of training in acute and chronic pain management beyond the physician's original certification in a subspecialty; only board-certified specialists can get this additional certificate. After this year of training, the physician must pass a written exam to receive the certificate. Two other bodies also offer additional certification in pain management: the American Board of Pain Medicine and the American Board of Pain Management.

- If you're looking for a pain management specialist, be sure she or he is board-certified in a primary specialty and also has additional training and experience in pain management.

The American Board of Medical Specialties is the oversight board for all specialty practices. Your physician should have a certificate from one of its members; to check this, call the board at (800) 776-2378 or visit its website at http://www.abms.org. For doctors not listed at this website, try the American Academy of Pain medicine website: www.painorg.com.

This new willingness and ability to treat chronic pain come at a time when 34 million people suffer from this condition. Indeed, according to the National Institute of Neurological Disorders and Stroke, chronic pain is the most expensive health problem in the country: health care expenses, lost workdays, compensation, and legal expenses add up to an annual cost of $50 billion.

More effective and widespread treatment of pain can also defuse the hotly debated issue of assisted suicide—for, as our ability to manage pain increases, the need for assisted suicide diminishes. Most of the people who ask for assistance in dying have severe, unrelenting chronic pain, and the main reason so many people believe that assisted suicide must be an option is that adequate pain treatment centers are not yet universally available. Even where such clinics exist, the physicians caring for people with chronic pain aren't always aware of them.

Another contributing factor to the debate is physicians' fear, mentioned above, that managing pain aggressively with narcotics will turn their patients into addicts. In my opinion, when the patient has a terminal illness, the doctor's attitude toward this question should be: "So what?" Although, as I've said, this fear is groundless in the first place, since most people don't become addicts.

The more effectively chronic pain can be treated, the less likely people will be to ask for assistance in dying. We can hope that, as pain clinics become more widely available, the need for this service will fade away.

Addiction Is Not a Big Risk

It's true that some people who receive narcotics from a physician—for example, after minor surgery—do become addicted and realize they can get more narcotics by continuing to have pain. For these people the primary problem is addiction, not pain; their psychological state is one of addiction, and pain happens to be the way to satisfy that addiction. Indeed, many people come to pain clinics simply to obtain their fix of narcotics. That is why these clinics screen prospective patients carefully to determine what their real problems are.

For the vast majority of people, however, the fear that taking narcotics will lead to addiction is groundless, based on a misunderstanding of the distinction between addiction and physical dependence. If you take a narcotic for longer than a few days, then stop taking it cold, without a tapering-off period, you are likely to have temporary nausea, chills, and muscle cramps. But this is quite different from the addict's craving for a high that leads to continued, self-destructive abuse of the drug.

Whereas an addict tends to require larger and larger doses of narcotics, a person who has real pain usually gets relief from continuing the same dose for a long period of time. Richard's infusion pump, for example, was set to deliver a specified dose that controlled his pain without needing to be increased. Over time, such a person may require slight elevations in the dose. But studies show that even though some people are susceptible to addiction, many of these don't become addicts, even when they receive narcotics. Out of twenty-five thousand cancer patients in three studies, only seven became addicted to narcotics.

One reason taking narcotics for pain does not create addiction is that the narcotics we give for chronic pain are slow-release drugs. They are absorbed by the body slowly, without giving you the kind of rush that addicts seek. "With addicts, their quality of life goes down as they use drugs," Dr. Scott Fishman, chief of the division of pain medicine at the University of California–Davis, explained to *New York* magazine. "With pain patients, it improves. They're entirely different phenomena."

When someone who does not have pain takes a narcotic, instead of being used to counteract the effects of pain, the drug will attach to specialized opiate receptors on nerve cells (narcotics are also called opiates since many derive from opium) and produce a high. What is more, new opiate receptors are induced that also require narcotics, causing the body to crave more narcotics. A vicious cycle develops, in which the craving intensifies until the patient is taken off narcotics entirely; when this is done, the number of receptors returns to normal.

This physiological mechanism explains why evaluation to discover the cause of your pain is critical: if the doctor can find a clear, identifiable cause, you are less likely to become an addict. Note that although Richard's doctors could not identify the precise cause of his pain—since chronic back pain is an extremely complex syndrome—it was clear that such a cause did exist. Thus Richard was in little danger of becoming addicted to the drugs he was receiving. Besides, my nephew was watching him closely for the telltale indication of addiction: that he was asking for higher doses of narcotic because his pain was no longer being relieved. If this happened, my nephew would tell him that he was in danger of becoming addicted and must try to cope with his current dosage level.

Complex Pain Syndromes

Unrelenting pain that lasts longer than six weeks can be considered chronic. Chronic pain syndromes occur frequently after traumatic injuries; after any kind of surgery; after illnesses that damage nerves, such as *herpes zoster* infection, AIDS, and diabetes; after certain drug treatments that also injure nerves (such as taking AZT for AIDS); and after invasion of nerves by cancer. Some forms of chronic pain result from the response of brain cells to changes in nerve impulses caused by the injuries listed above. One example is phantom limb pain, which involves feeling persistent and sometimes severe pain in an arm or leg that has been amputated. Sometimes no specific cause for chronic pain can be found, as in Richard's case.

Whatever the reason for pain, there's no value in the notion that people should simply learn to cope with it. Research has revealed that the entire brain—not just one part of it, as previously thought—responds to pain. Not only does pain dominate the brain, making the person unable to pay attention to other input, but it can actually rewire the nervous system pathways in such a way that the pain spreads to other parts of the body. You should therefore make sure your pain is treated early, before these permanent changes have time to develop.

When chronic pain occurs, additional factors usually affect the patient's response to it. Frequently—and understandably—people become depressed. They are exhausted because they can't sleep and either lose or gain weight. The experience of pain also affects relationships with family and friends; for example, some people find that pain earns them attention they wouldn't receive otherwise. For others, particularly manual laborers, the response to pain may be related to unpleasant working conditions. Around the age of forty, when the body starts to wear out, some begin to feel as though life would be easier if they could be declared disabled and receive workers' compensation. On top of these psychological issues, many people in pain have been treated by their primary care doctors with a variety of drugs, including narcotics and sedatives, without evaluation of the additional effects of depression. This can lead to a worsening of their overall condition.

For all these reasons, we don't speak simply of chronic pain but rather of complex chronic pain syndromes. This term refers not only to the pain itself but to the many associated problems that accompany it. Pain syndromes are treated most successfully in a multidisciplinary setting.

The Multidisciplinary Approach

Many pain clinics combine several fields of practice into a team approach. The International Association for the Study of Pain describes four types of facility:

Modality-oriented clinics offer one specific treatment, such as nerve blocks, biofeedback, or acupuncture.

Pain clinics specialize in diagnosing and treating chronic pain, sometimes focusing on specific diagnoses or parts of the body.

Multidisciplinary pain clinics also diagnose and treat chronic pain, but their staffs include physicians from different specialties as well as other personnel, such as nurses, occupational therapists, and acupuncturists.

Multidisciplinary pain centers, in addition to treatment staff, also have staff devoted to teaching and research.

Like every other field of medicine, pain management has been affected by the growth of HMOs. In the 1980s chronic pain patients typically spent six to eight weeks as inpatients in pain clinics. Today outpatient care is the norm. What's more, most people have difficulty getting effective treatment for chronic pain because insurance companies, and especially Medicaid and Medicare, often won't reimburse for it. This reluctance is probably due to the fact that chronic pain management requires many time-consuming visits, as well as the use of new and expensive modalities, which may be experimental and lack outcome data to support their effectiveness (although the results of smaller studies that have been done are very encouraging).

Typically, a pain facility will want to see your medical records before accepting you as a patient; some will only accept patients referred by health professionals. You may first be screened by a psychologist, who administers personality tests to unearth any problems that indicate malingering or other disorders, such as depression, anxiety, or hysteria. These could interfere psychologically with relief of pain. Someone who is addicted to narcotics must be treated for addiction before their pain can be relieved.

After psychological testing, you're seen by a pain specialist, who is often an anesthesiologist but can also be a neurosurgeon, physiatrist (rehabilitation specialist), neurologist, or internist. This doctor begins to focus on your pain complaint. After looking for the cause, he or she initiates treatment. For example, a patient with facial pain may have a recent history of scabs and sores on the face. This alerts the pain specialist that the patient has a postherpetic syndrome, and treatment is chosen accordingly.

During this process, other team members can be called in. An internist is available to manage the medications you are currently taking and help select additional ones. A neurologist and neurosurgeon will evaluate problems that may require surgery. A social worker assesses your family dynamics and works with your family during your treatment. An occupational therapist helps you handle disabilities the pain may have caused; for example, a painful arm being treated with nerve blocks can improve further with various exercises that the therapist teaches you. At some point the entire team gets together to discuss your treatment as a whole.

Since you are dealing with a chronic condition, treatment can last for years. Unfortunately, in most cases the doctor is unable to make chronic pain go away completely, although the multidisciplinary approach can help people moderate the experience by teaching them to cope with pain more effectively. Often, however, patients wind up going from clinic to clinic seeking relief. I realize it's frustrating when treatments don't work, but if your doctor knows your condition and you've researched all aspects of your diagnosis, chances are that you won't achieve much by going elsewhere. In fact, another doctor might only add to your unhappiness by giving you more medications without discontinuing your previous ones. And if you persist in an endless search for a new doctor, you risk ending up with a quack who could do you more harm than good.

Physicians, for their part, frequently become discouraged too when they can't provide complete pain relief, especially since pain patients tend to be quite demanding. Their desperation drives them to call and insist on talking with the doctor, who may have nothing more to offer, and to make frequent appointments, which are likely to turn into therapy sessions instead of medical treatment.

- If you're struggling with chronic pain and have generally been happy with your physician, try to remember that she or he may indeed be doing all that can be done.

Chronic Pain Conditions

Our greatest successes in treating chronic pain come primarily with cancer pain and with low back pain that hasn't been relieved by surgery. Patients with other types of chronic pain, as I noted, often can't obtain complete relief. These are the desperate souls who wind up trying one doctor after another.

Low Back Pain

Low back pain is the most common complaint that brings people to pain clinics. Since pain fibers exist in most of the structures of the low back, a variety of injuries to the muscles or ligaments can cause low back pain. So can degeneration of the spine due to osteoporosis. The cause that most frequently brings people in for treatment of low back pain is a slipped disk, which causes pain by pressing on the nerves as they exit the spinal canal.

When we find a cause of low back pain, we can treat it specifically— by surgically removing a slipped disk, for example. Frequently, however, no cause can be found. In such a case we may try medications, including nonsteroidal anti-inflammatory drugs (NSAIDs), antidepressants (since pain is closely related to a person's psychological state, sometimes antidepressants relieve it), drugs that block the sympathetic nervous system (which maintains a state of excitation), and tranquilizers. We try these drugs in various combinations and doses until adequate pain relief—or as much as possible—is achieved. If none of these medications are effective, as a last resort we will give narcotics, either orally or in patches. In the process, we must balance the side effects of the drugs against the degree of pain relief they provide. If, for example, nausea and vomiting from drugs limit someone's ability to function, that's not much of an improvement in the person's life.

Another possibility, when no abnormality can be identified as the cause, is to give a diagnostic nerve block by injecting either a local anesthetic or a steroid drug—or a combination of both—around the nerve, to see if the pain stops. Often after two or three of these blocks, the pain will disappear for six or eight months. Subsequent injections may be necessary, although generally the intervals between them grow longer.

Patients who have had multiple back operations, whose pain persists even though no abnormality can be found, may be helped by an intrathecal catheter like the one Richard received or by a spinal cord stimulator, which produces a low electric current that sends pain-inhibiting impulses to the spinal cord. Unfortunately, these two methods relieve intractable low back pain in only 50 to 75 percent of patients. But without treatment, the success rate is zero. So if previous back surgery has been unsuccessful, this is certainly an option to try.

Postherpetic Neuralgia

Some people who contract an infection with *herpes zoster* (the virus that causes chickenpox) develop severe pain, called postherpetic neuralgia or shingles, in affected nerves in the skin after the infection is over. The skin areas over the course of the affected nerves are hypersensitive to any stimulation, such as the touch of clothing, and painful even in the absence of stimulation. Postherpetic syndrome that occurs in the trigeminal nerve,

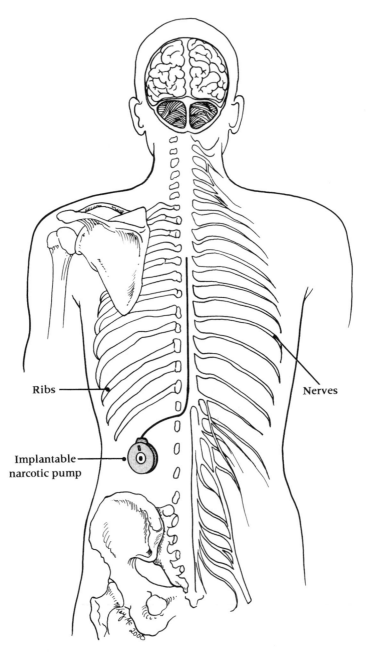

Ribs

Nerves

Implantable
narcotic pump

Fig. 18. Intrathecal implantable narcotic pump for relief of chronic pain. An implanted spinal cord stimulator would be placed beneath the skin at the same location, with two wire electrodes threaded through catheters running on both sides of the spinal cord.

which supplies the face, is one cause of the excruciating facial pain known as trigeminal neuralgia or tic douloureux.

As soon as a skin eruption on your face or chest is diagnosed as a herpes infection, you should immediately begin treatment to avoid development of severe pain. This treatment consists of blocks of the involved nerves, which seem to preempt the onset of chronic pain after the infection. If treatment is not initiated early, patients often develop severe pain that can't be relieved.

For patients who haven't had this initial treatment and do develop severe pain, we first try diagnostic nerve blocks with local anesthetics. These sometimes relieve pain for about six hours. If we try these blocks two or three times but the pain continues to return, we need to consider intrathecal drugs, spinal cord stimulation, radiofrequency ablation, or cryotherapy.

Radiofrequency ablation has become increasingly popular. We place a wire around the area of the nerve causing pain, then use an external computer to send radiofrequency signals to the nerve, creating heat. The heat "stuns" the nerve, interrupting the pain signal. It's like unplugging a lamp, since the nerve is still intact and eventually will regenerate and be plugged back in. For this reason, in most cases the procedure must be repeated every six to twenty-four months.

Cryotherapy is similar. We place a probe in the area of the nerve causing pain and use a computer to create an "ice ball" around the nerve. Like heat, freezing stuns the nerve. It works quite well, but unfortunately must often be repeated monthly because the effects are short-lived.

We use permanent blocks only rarely, for they have serious drawbacks. They create permanent numbness and may impair movement. After a block has been given, pain can return with greater intensity; this is called "deafferentation syndrome."

Postherpetic neuralgias are indeed very difficult to treat.

- If you develop a herpes zoster infection, be sure to ask for nerve blocks immediately.
- If you do develop severe postherpetic pain, ask for radiofrequency ablation or cryotherapy.

A new option for treating postherpetic pain is a patch approved by the Food and Drug Administration in 1999. The patch contains a solution of lidocaine, a local anesthetic, in a form that penetrates the skin sufficiently to affect the nerves. Studies showed that the patch was effective for 60 to 70 percent of the relatively small number of patients who tried it.

Sometimes tic douloureux (trigeminal neuralgia) develops without previous signs or symptoms of herpetic infection. It's been suggested that in such a case the pain is caused by compression of the trigeminal nerve inside the skull by a pulsating blood vessel or other structure. If all other treatments fail, we can perform intracranial surgery to identify structures that may be pressing on the nerve and relieve the pressure. Even this procedure, however, is still only about 50 to 60 percent effective.

- If you have tic douloureux that can't be relieved, see a neurosurgeon; he or she may be able to relieve your pain.

Postinjury Pain

Severe injury to an arm or a leg may lead to a postinjury pain syndrome caused by damage to the sympathetic nervous system in that part of the body. People experience burning pain in the limb, as well as skin changes resulting in loss of hair. After surgery for a back injury sustained in a car accident, one man suffered continual pain in his legs due to nerve damage in his back. "I can't shower because the water feels like molten lava," he told a reporter for *U.S. News and World Report.* "Every time someone turns on a ceiling fan, it feels like razor blades are cutting through my legs." At thirty-five, he had been to twenty doctors and was contemplating suicide.

In the past, postinjury pain was divided into two categories: sympathetic dystrophy and causalgia. These terms referred to, respectively, less severe and more severe burning pain in a part of the body supplied by a nerve that had been injured. Because of their essential similarities, these two conditions are now both known as complex regional pain syndrome.

The treatment for this syndrome is a block of the sympathetic nervous system, which controls the tone of blood vessels. Pain may be the result of blood vessel spasm, which causes ischemia (decreased blood supply), which in turn leads to pain. The block allows the vessels to relax so that more blood can flow into the painful area, thereby decreasing the pain. In addition to changing the blood flow, sympathetic blocks often result in a "calming down" of the sympathetic nerve fibers. These two processes work hand in hand to reduce pain. Initially, blocks are done diagnostically; when repeated, they may or may not relieve the pain for long periods. Here we must consider alternatives: intrathecal infusions and spinal stimulation.

For pain in the arms and hands, we block the stellate ganglion, a mass of nerve cells at the side of the neck. Because this ganglion is close to important structures, performing the block risks serious complications. One is seizures. Another is what we call "total spinal," in which the local anesthetic goes into the spinal canal and causes hypotension and cessation of breathing. A third is that the block can affect the nerve for speech, paralyzing the vocal cord on the involved side of the body and causing permanent hoarseness. Still another possibility is Horner's syndrome, a condition in which damage to a cervical nerve affects the eye, causing the eyeball to sink inward and the upper eyelid to droop, among other changes.

We can also treat arm pain with an intrathecal catheter, placing the catheter in the lower neck and infusing clonidine, a sympatholytic drug (one that blocks sympathetic nerve impulses); local anesthetics; or narcotics.

For leg and foot pain, we give lumbar epidurals, using local anesthetics to block the sympathetic nervous system. If repeated epidurals are effective, you should consider having a permanent infusion pump implanted that would continuously infuse a local anesthetic, a narcotic, or clonidine.

Cancer Pain

You should know that patients who suffer from cancer pain no longer need to take large doses of oral narcotics. We now have treatments that offer significant relief without the adverse side effects of these drugs.

One alternative is diagnostic nerve blocks followed by permanent blocks. Pain in the upper gastrointestinal tract caused by cancer of the pancreas, stomach, gallbladder, or liver is successfully treated by blocking the celiac plexus (a mass of nerves lying in the center of the trunk, just below the stomach). This block should be done under fluoroscopy, especially if a permanent block is being performed after successful diagnostic blocks. A permanent block can provide pain relief for up to six months.

Pain from cervical, ovarian, and uterine cancer is often treated with an epidural injection of narcotics. We can implant an infusion pump that gives relief for the rest of the patient's life. Another possibility is a diagnostic intrathecal injection of narcotics. If this is successful, and the pain is severe, we can consider a permanent neurolytic block. You should be aware, however, that the potential side effects of this block include loss of bowel and bladder control, as well as muscle weakness in the legs that could impair walking.

Pain from tumors of the head and neck is commonly treated with a stellate ganglion block. Again, we can do this first diagnostically, then, if the patient so decides, administer a permanent block. Lung cancer, breast cancer, and other cancers that cause chest wall pain can be relieved by an epidural around the spinal canal. We can also place intrathecal catheters inside the spinal canal. Occasionally, a catheter may be inserted directly into the pleural space (between the two parts of the pleura, the membrane that lines the lungs and the inner wall of the chest cavity), although this is not commonly done. Through each of these catheters, we administer a combination of local anesthetics and narcotics.

An important point about diagnostic blocks: your cooperation is absolutely necessary in order for the pain specialist to correctly identify the affected nerve. These blocks are often painful, but if you ask for too much sedation and analgesia, it will not be possible to tell whether the block is working. When it's placed correctly, you experience almost immediate relief. The way for the doctor to know this is for you to be awake to report your sensations as the block is being placed.

A final option for cancer pain relief is antidepressant drugs. Some people are reluctant to take them because they don't want others to think they're "crazy." But if you have a life-threatening, chronic disease, you have good reason to be depressed, and if that's the case, these drugs can actually alter your perception of pain.

- Don't refuse antidepressants if your physician suggests them.

Neck Pain

Neck pain caused by whiplash and sports injuries can also be successfully treated. For pain in the back of the neck, we give local nerve blocks. If these are unsuccessful, we give a cervical epidural, which is very effective, especially for whiplash injury.

Headaches

Mary came to an emergency room complaining of the worst headache she'd ever had, pulsating behind one eye. It was so bad that she'd become nauseous and vomited. What brought her to the ER, explained Mary, who was forty-four, was having read descriptions of the symptoms of stroke; she feared she was having one. But after taking a detailed history, giving her a thorough examination, and taking her blood pressure, the doctor ruled this out. Mary's sister and grandmother, it seemed, had experienced similar headaches, sometimes lasting for days; this history, together with her symptoms, led him to conclude that in fact, she was having a migraine. Just to be sure, he sent her for a CAT scan to definitively rule out stroke and brain tumor.

Next he asked what had been happening to her lately. Mary had recently lost her job; the resulting distress led her to drink more coffee than usual. Immediately before the migraine began, she'd been drinking red wine and eating cheese. As it happens, migraine tends to occur in people with acute anxiety or depression, as well as in susceptible people who consume large amounts of caffeine or eat foods like cheese and wine that are rich in histamine-producing substances (that is, which provoke allergic reactions). People who take vasodilator drugs for heart disease and women who take contraceptive pills or postmenopausal hormone replacement therapy are also at risk for migraine.

Migraine, though excruciating, is only one type of headache, and not even the worst. Indeed, headaches are a way of life in America today. The most common types are classified into five main categories: migraine, cluster, tension, posttraumatic, and infectious.

Migraines

The French philosopher Simone Weil, who suffered from agonizing migraine headaches from 1930, when she was twenty-one, until her death in 1943, wrote of "the terrible temptation I feel when my courage gives out, to use my headaches as an alibi, an excuse for my idleness and all my failings." Forbidding herself to succumb to that temptation, she taught classes, read voluminously, and wrote countless articles and essays through a fog of pain. In fact, she wound up constructing an entire social philosophy on the experience of pain, which she transformed into a path to salvation.[1]

Most migraine sufferers don't find salvation in their headaches, but frequent pain may indeed lead them to forgo many of life's pleasures as well as its responsibilities. Migraines are worse than common tension headaches. Typically, they begin with a premonitory experience called an aura, which usually consists of visual abnormalities called scotomas. These include both blind spots and hallucinations of brilliant, scintillating shapes, such as herringbone zigzags, whorls, and lattices. Shortly after, the headache starts behind one eye, though not always the same eye. Some sufferers have migraines as often as several times a week; others only twice a year. The frequency tends to diminish with age.

Migraine seems to occur when blood vessels in the brain constrict in response to triggering factors, such as those responsible for Mary's headache: stress, anxiety, caffeine, and certain foods, as well as dehydration. After the vasoconstriction phase, the vessels dilate, resulting in increased pressure inside the skull that produces the headache. The first measure in preventing migraine, therefore, is to avoid triggering behaviors and substances (you need to find out which ones particularly affect you). Psychological help in relieving stress-related anxiety, as well as relaxation techniques like biofeedback, are somewhat effective. Acupuncture (see the section describing it below) is also helpful, though not consistently, and its effects seem not to last after the treatments stop. Drugs are the most effective treatment; in fact, major advances were made in the 1990s in developing drugs specifically to treat migraine.

After other causes have been ruled out, as with Mary, drug treatment of migraine is geared toward disrupting the cycle of vasoconstriction followed by vasodilation. One preventive measure is to give a beta blocker, such as propranolol, to keep the vessels from constricting in the first place. Beta blockers can decrease the frequency of attacks. After the headache has already developed, drugs that enhance certain actions of the neurotransmitter serotonin can relieve pain, since serotonin can act as a vasoconstrictor or vasodilator. A variety of these serotonin agonists are available, including sumatriptan, naratriptan, and rizatriptan. Some work for some people, others for other people; your doctor will try first the one that works on the largest number. These drugs can be taken orally, nasally, rectally, or by intramuscular injection. Since they are often poorly absorbed when taken orally, a subcutaneous injection might be more effective; in fact, we often give these drugs both orally and by injection to get rid of a headache. Studies have found that serotonin agonists are at least 70 percent effective in relieving migraine pain, with over 50 percent of sufferers achieving complete relief.

If you're among the 30 percent for whom these drugs don't work, we can try still another: dihydroergotamine, which combines the serotonin agonist effect with other mechanisms to cause vasoconstriction. If this doesn't work either, we must resort to older therapies: NSAIDs and possibly narcotics during acute attacks.

- Caution: If you have frequent migraines that are induced by
  stress, and you take narcotics for them, you risk developing
  a pattern of subconsciously getting a migraine in order to
  obtain narcotics and thereby becoming dependent on them.

It's best to avoid narcotics unless your pain is totally unbearable and completely unrelieved by any other measures.

Cluster Headaches

Cluster headaches are less common than migraines, but for people who have them, they generally occur more frequently than migraines, usually in the same location, and the pain can be more severe. Alcohol and vasodilator drugs are two triggering agents. Symptoms specific to these headaches include a stuffy nose and a red, tearing eye on the side of the headache. Cluster headaches occur in bouts; the headache lasts for about an hour, then disappears for half an hour, then returns in the same location. Whereas a migraine can last three days, a cluster headache lasts two to three hours.

Cluster headaches may be treated like migraines, by injection of sumatriptan. This measure is effective in about 75 percent of cases. Calcium channel blockers, which prevent spasm of the blood vessels, have been used, sometimes in combination with lithium, to decrease the frequency of bouts of cluster headaches. Prednisone, a corticosteroid, can also diminish the frequency of these headaches, but since it has adverse side effects, it should be taken only sparingly. If these measures all fail, we try the other triptans, dihydroergotamine, NSAIDs, and if absolutely necessary narcotics, as for migraine.

- If the initial treatment given you for cluster headaches fails, don't hesitate to ask for other types of drugs.
- If you're taking beta blockers, remember that these drugs can make you feel tired and decrease your sexual desire.

Tension Headache

This familiar type of headache, characterized by a dull pain or a feeling of tightness or pressure, usually on both sides of the head, can occur daily. Unlike migraines or cluster headaches, tension headaches don't involve visual abnormalities, nausea, or vomiting, and there's no typical duration. However, chronic tension headache frequently makes people unable to carry out their normal daily activities, so it can be as disabling as migraine.

We don't know what mechanism causes tension headaches; there's no evidence for vascular causes, as with migraine. A significant number of people who get them are depressed, however, and psychological tests suggest that tension headache is connected to anxiety, suppressed anger, and hypochondria as well. Muscle contraction in the neck, face, and head—such as a clenched jaw—can add to the headache's intensity.

Treatment starts with a complete work-up to rule out serious underlying causes. Stress-relief measures, such as psychological counseling and biofeedback, may ease the pain, as may acupuncture, antidepressant drugs, and NSAIDs. Serotonin agonists and the other drugs used for migraine and cluster headaches are not effective for tension headaches.

Posttraumatic Headache

Headache can result from head and neck injuries, such as whiplash. Injury to muscles, ligaments, or even bones that creates tension during head and neck movement may lead to pain. We can try a variety of techniques to treat posttraumatic headache: relaxation methods, such as guided imagery and progressive relaxation; NSAIDs; and muscle relaxants.

If all else fails, we use nerve blocks. Blocks of the occipital nerves affect the area running from behind the ear to the back and top of the head. We can also block nerves in the back of the neck and the base of the skull. Sometimes the pain is caused by vertebrae pressing on nerves, creating muscle tension that causes neck stiffness that then results in a headache. In such a case, we can prevent this entire cascade of events and virtually eliminate the headache by performing what are called facet blocks, which affect the surfaces where individual neck vertebrae articulate with each other.

A slipped cervical disk is another possible cause of posttraumatic headache. Often we can treat it successfully with a cervical epidural.

Infectious Headaches

When your sinuses are infected and blocked, you can develop a headache, often localized over the sinus, which feels tender to the touch. Treatment consists of antihistamines to relieve the blockage, antibiotics to resolve the infection, and NSAIDs to relieve the pain.

Temporomandibular Joint Disorder

Pain in the temporomandibular joint (TMJ), the hinge of the jaw, occurs most often after dental procedures or infection of the back teeth that spreads to the joint. Another possible cause is an injury, such as a blow to the head or neck. TMJ pain occurs in front of or behind the ear and can radiate anywhere over that side of the face. Often sensation in the painful area is diminished. Frequently, the person clenches the jaw, which makes the pain worse. TMJ is often misdiagnosed as trigeminal neuralgia; it's important to be sure which condition you have, since the treatments are different.

Treating TMJ disorder requires careful adjustment of the bite by a dental surgeon, along with biofeedback and other therapies to reduce the clenching of the jaw muscles. As a last resort, we can do a block of the auriculotemporal nerve, which runs up the face in front of the ear, although this is not always effective.

Pain Treatment Modalities

This section further elaborates on treatment methods referred to above and describes new ones.

Transcutaneous Electrical Stimulation (TENS)

TENS is a form of electrical stimulation that uses an external device about the size of a cigarette pack that is placed on the skin surface. A set of electrodes running from it are attached to the skin by a conducting paste. The stimulator generates a series of pulses whose intensity and frequency can be adjusted until you feel a tingling sensation in the painful area. We think that this stimulation inhibits the spinal cord cells that transmit pain messages to the brain. TENS doesn't usually work for moderate or severe pain, but can be effective for mild pain, as from a mild form of postherpetic neuralgia.

Drug Cocktails

Patients with chronic pain are often taking a "drug cocktail," which consists of several different types of compounds that affect different pain channels. Typically, a drug cocktail includes an antidepressant, a sedative, a narcotic, and an anticonvulsant drug. The anticonvulsant—the same type of drug used for epilepsy—is thought to prevent transmission of pain impulses by stabilizing the nerve cell membranes.

The Latest Techniques

One brand-new way to deliver narcotics is a lollipop infused with narcotics. When you suck on it, the drugs are absorbed by the mucous lining of the inside of the cheek and sent directly into the bloodstream. You experience the effects almost as rapidly as with intravenous morphine. Equally remarkable is a newly developed morphine inhaler, which works even faster.

An Ancient Technique: Acupuncture

Acupuncture is a two-thousand-year-old Chinese practice in which needles as fine as a hair are inserted into points on the body that lie along pathways of energy flow. The Chinese explanation is that the needles restore this energy flow in areas where it is blocked. Western researchers have suggested that the needles elicit the release of endorphins, naturally occurring narcotics, which relieve the pain. The amount of endorphins released depends on genetics; for example, people of Asian descent seem to respond with a greater release of endorphins than Caucasians. Thus, whereas acupuncture is effective among Westerners largely for pain that is less than moderate, it may be effective in other cultures even for moderate pain.

In 1997 acupuncture was endorsed by a panel convened by the National Institutes of Health, which concluded that it was effective for nausea and vomiting resulting from cancer chemotherapy, pregnancy, or surgical anesthesia, and for pain after dental surgery. The panel added that it might also work for menstrual cramps, fibromyalgia (a generalized muscle pain), stroke, headache, and tennis elbow. Testimony from people who try it often goes further. In 1998 *Health* magazine described Catherine, a woman left in terrible pain after a car accident, who tried acupuncture only because she was desperate. She went to her first appointment in a highly skeptical frame of mind, but found that the treatment was successful where drugs and physical therapy hadn't been: while not completely healed, within a few months she was back riding her horse and living a normal life.

Catherine is a typical pain patient, whose story demonstrates how subjective an experience pain is. The perception of pain depends on several factors, for example, the amount of circulating stress hormones (epinephrine or noradrenaline) in relation to endorphins. Acupuncture worked for Catherine, while someone else might only find relief from invasive resection of a nerve. Some people have knee or hip replacements because of joint pain; for others acupuncture takes care of it. So if you have chronic pain, it's important to be willing to try anything, no matter how little faith you might have in some techniques, for truly—and I say this as a doctor—you never know.

- If you are planning a strategy for treating chronic pain, start with the least invasive methods first.

The two exceptions here are a slipped disk and postherpetic neuralgia. For these conditions, you need to begin with a more invasive treatment, such as epidural steroids or intercostal nerve blocks.

Resources for Coping with Chronic Pain

American Academy of Pain Management
13947 Mono Way #A
Sonora CA 95370.
Phone: (209) 533-9744
E-mail: aapm@aapainmanage.org
Website: www.aapainmanage.org

American Chronic Pain Association
257 Old Haymaker Rd.
Monroeville, PA 15146
Phone: (412) 856-9676
Fax: (916) 632-3208.
E-mail: ACPA@pacbell.net
Website: www.theacpa.org

American Pain Society
4700 W. Lake Avenue
Glenview, IL 60025
Phone: (847) 375-4715
Fax: (847) 375-6315
E-mail: info@ampainsoc.org
Website: www.ampainsoc.org

American Society of Anesthesiology
520 Northwest Highway
Park Ridge, IL 60068
Phone: (847) 825-5586
Fax: (847) 825-1692
Website: www.asahq.org
Education, Patient Education Brochures, Management of Pain

National Chronic Pain Outreach Association (NCPOA)
7979 Old Georgetown Road, Suite 100
Bethesda, MD 20814-2429
Phone: (301) 652-4948
Fax: (301) 907-0745
Website: http://neurosurgery.mgh.harvard.edu/NCPAINOA.HTM

Summary: Questions and Points to Remember

- In discussing your pain with your doctor, refer to the clinical practice guidelines issued by the Agency for Health Care Policy and Research as an appropriate standard for your care.
- If you're looking for a pain management specialist, be sure she or he is board-certified in a primary specialty and also has additional training and experience in pain management.
- If you're struggling with chronic pain and have generally been happy with your physician, try to remember that he or she may indeed be doing all that can be done.
- If you develop a herpes zoster infection, be sure to ask for nerve blocks immediately.
- If you do develop severe postherpetic pain, ask for radio-frequency ablation or cryotherapy.
- If you have tic douloureux that can't be relieved, see a neurosurgeon; she or he may be able to relieve your pain.
- Don't refuse antidepressants as a treatment for cancer pain if your physician suggests them.
- Caution: If you have frequent migraines that are induced by stress, and you take narcotics for them, you risk developing a pattern of subconsciously getting a migraine in order to obtain narcotics and thereby becoming dependent on them.
- If the initial treatment given you for cluster headaches fails, don't hesitate to ask for other types of drugs.
- If you're taking beta blockers for headache, remember that these drugs can make you feel tired and decrease your sexual desire.
- If you are planning a strategy for treating chronic pain, start with the least invasive methods first, except in cases of slipped disk and postherpetic neuralgia.

NOTE

1. Stephanie Golden, *Slaying the Mermaid: Women and the Culture of Sacrifice* (New York: Harmony Books, 1998), 196.

• • •

CHAPTER 17

The Future of Anesthesia

• • •

In 1977, when Sally was almost twelve, she had her tonsils out. The tonsils were huge, and her pediatrician felt that if they ever became swollen, her already small air passage might narrow further and create a breathing problem. Sally herself wanted the procedure because she hoped it would put an end to the teasing she endured over her snoring, both from her sister at home and at sleep-away camp.

Her mother took her to a well-known, quite elderly doctor who performed tonsillectomies out of a big old house in Brooklyn, set up with a surgery and recovery area. "I remember very vividly being wide awake, strapped on a gurney in the OR," Sally told me.

There were two nurses on either side of me, and the doctor was at my feet. The medical team might have told me what was going to happen next, but I don't recall that. I only remember a mask with a cold metal rim going over my nose and mouth, and I smelled the most thick and noxious fume I had ever encountered. I completely panicked and started moving my head furiously. As they tried to put the mask over my nose and mouth again, I began screaming for my mother and thrashing my body and feet so that the gurney would move. I remember the doctor admonishing me to stop kicking and that my mother would be angry at how I was behaving. I was really begging them to stop, saying I couldn't breathe.

Finally, a heavyset nurse to my right leaned over and lay over my chest to keep the gurney from shifting. Her weight was crushing me, and I was crying for her to get off. From somewhere came the mask again, held firm and tight over my nose and mouth. The air was so thick, my throat burned, and I truly felt like I was going to die. The last thing I remember was hearing this ringing sound that got louder and louder, and then everything blacked out.

Meanwhile, the staff told Sally's mother to call her father. Since most children came out of anesthesia fighting, the way they went under, they said she would need help when Sally awoke.

Not surprisingly, this experience left Sally (much like Aaron Beck, described in chapter 1) with a long-standing terror of strong smells.

> If I was in an elevator and someone walked in wearing a strong perfume or cologne, I became anxious. At a gas station, the smell of the gasoline sent me into a near panic. When I was about thirteen, I was in a small pinball arcade with a few friends. Some kids threw in a few smoke bombs and shut the door with us inside. As the room filled with smoke and the air became quite thick, I freaked out, screaming and crying and banging my hands against the windows and the doors. When I finally got out, I was in pretty bad shape. And there was no consoling me. It was awful.
>
> Needless to say, for many years I was terrified of having to undergo surgery. Even at the dentist, I took the drilling straight, with no sweet air or Novocain. I wanted to be wide awake and in control.

Even for 1977, Sally's experience was unusually gruesome—not representative of standard anesthesia practice. But it does illustrate how far patient comfort has come: today we don't use a mask; we give children sedatives; and we don't hold them down, because we don't have to. As this book has explained, anesthesia today is far more patient-friendly than it used to be. For children in particular, the involvement of parents up to the moment of induction, as well as the use of new drugs that provide effective sedation and a gentler induction, has made the kind of nightmare that Sally suffered through a thing of the past.

And in the future, things will get even better. So in concluding this book, I'd like to speculate on upcoming developments in anesthesiology.

Increasing the Safety of Anesthesia

Although Sally's tonsillectomy was successful and ended safely, her terror was in fact justified, for her life was certainly threatened by the nurse leaning on her chest as the ether mask was placed over her face. As you may recall from the story in chapter 6 of the three-hundred-pound woman who nearly died during childbirth, ether was difficult to administer safely. With someone putting pressure on her chest and abdomen, Sally could have aspirated stomach contents into her lungs, or stopped breathing entirely.

At that time, too, there were no standard safety guidelines. The subsequent development of such guidelines has substantially improved the safety of anesthesia, and the future promises even greater progress. In 1984 the Anesthesia Patient Safety Foundation (www.gasnet.org/apsf) was created specifically to recommend clinical standards for all patients receiving anesthesia. These guidelines described what monitors and other standards of practice were appropriate for different medical conditions. Thus, if a patient suffered a cardiac arrest after a failed intubation, for example, and an end-tidal carbon dioxide monitor hadn't been used, that could be considered malpractice.

In 1999 the Institute of Medicine (the medical branch of the National Academy of Sciences) issued a report stating that physicians' errors resulted in forty-four thousand to ninety-eight thousand deaths per year. Repeatedly, this report alluded to the progress in patient safety that had been made in anesthesiology, in contrast to other fields of medicine—progress due to the creation of these clinical guidelines and to better monitoring of vital signs. The Institute report recommended that all medical disciplines institute a similar system.

Whereas before the Anesthesia Patient Safety Foundation was created, there was about 1 death for every 4,000 times that anesthesia was given, today this figure is about 1 in 250,000. And in the future, we hope it will be close to zero. Several upcoming developments in medicine—and in anesthesia in particular—give this hope a solid basis in reality.

First, much like airline pilots using simulators to learn to manage flight emergencies, future anesthesiologists in training will practice correcting apnea and sudden swings in blood pressure and heart rate that can occur during surgery, using computers and mannequins that actually simulate patients with complex medical problems receiving anesthesia. Training will also cover low-frequency disasters like allergic reactions to latex gloves.

Second, other innovations under development will allow us to prevent these abnormalities from occurring in the first place. Artificial blood substitutes that remain in the circulation long enough to be used during surgery hold promise of avoiding life-threatening reactions to transfusions of real blood. Electrical devices that detect—and correct—heart arrhythmias as they occur may make cardiac arrest under anesthesia a thing of the past. And researchers are working on a way to minimize the damage caused by a stroke that occurs during surgery and anesthesia. For example, lack of oxygen during surgery for aneurysm or arteriovenous malformations can damage brain tissue. But within the mitochondria, tiny structures inside the nerve cells, there are genes that control the production of proteins created in response to stress that help repair damaged tissue. We expect to be able to stimulate these genes in advance to produce those proteins before or during the operation itself, thereby preventing permanent neurological injury. The stimulator could be an anesthetic, some other type of drug, or an electrical stimulus.

Third, medical control of certain diseases will also contribute to decreasing mortality during anesthesia. For example, a cure for sickle cell disease—again using genetic alterations—is just on the horizon. Since patients with sickle cell disease are more likely to have stroke, renal failure, and heart attack under anesthesia than other people, curing their disease will make anesthesia safer for them. Alternatively, a new inhaled gas, nitric oxide, can prevent these complications by dilating the blood vessels, thereby avoiding the insufficient oxygen supply that causes the higher risk in the first place.

Finally, the future will bring new artificial organs, light and unobtrusive, that can be attached and worn outside the body, making many types of invasive transplant surgery, with their attendant anesthetic risks, unnecessary.

New Ways to Deliver Anesthesia

Much research is now underway to define precisely how anesthetics actually cause analgesia. Once we discover the secret of these basic mechanisms, we can figure out different methods for initiating anesthesia. Perhaps it will be possible to interrupt nerve impulses with a magnetic or electrical signal, instead of a drug. Then we could induce anesthesia far more simply, by placing an electrode into the area that will cause the pain—or on the skin over that area—and then delivering an electric current through the electrode or creating a magnetic field to interrupt the pain signal traveling through the nerves.

Another proposed technique to interrupt pain transmission is a feedback delivery system that measures levels of prostaglandins and substance P, pain-inducing hormones in the blood that are produced in response to tissue damage. Researchers are working to develop drugs that can neutralize the effects of these pain hormones. Delivering these drugs via an infusion pump can, again, effectively prevent the perception of pain.

Molecular biology may hold other answers to the problem of decreasing pain transmission during surgery. One possibility is stimulating genes to rapidly produce antipain substances, such as endorphins. Another is identifying ways to use blood electrolytes to create anesthetic effects. For example, lithium, an ion similar to sodium, functions as an electrolyte and is currently given for bipolar disorder. It works by interfering with the absorption of sodium by nerves, decreasing the transmission of certain impulses into the brain and ultimately boosting the production of feel-good hormones like the neurotransmitter serotonin. The effect of these changes is to calm the person down during the manic phase of the disorder. If we developed an ion with similar actions that we could infuse during surgery, we could similarly interfere with the effects of pain-causing substances that are released—an easy way to deliver anesthesia.

Yet another possibility is the anticipated development of anesthetic drugs that selectively affect just the dorsal horn (an area of the spinal cord that sends pain signals to the brain), thereby avoiding unwanted blocking of sympathetic or motor nerves.

Noninvasive Surgery

As surgery becomes increasingly noninvasive, surgical pain may diminish and with it, the need for anesthesia. Take the history of treatment for kidney stones, for example. In the past, the stones were removed by open surgery, which created a great deal of pain both during and after the operation. Today the stones are often removed using sound waves, and pain is much less severe.

Similarly, prostate surgery is currently being done experimentally through a transrectal (through the rectum) ultrasound approach. An ultrasound device locates the prostate, allowing a laser to be guided into the area to vaporize the diseased tissue. Other uses of ultrasound allow transrectal delivery of hyperthermia (heat) to a diseased area. A probe is inserted under ultrasound guidance to destroy the tissue by heating it. The use of ultrasound to locate prostate cancer through the urethra, in order to treat it with cryosurgery—that is, destroying the tissue with extreme cold—is also being studied.

As we saw, laser surgery, laparoscopic surgery both with and without lasers (particularly for gallbladder removal), and advances in interventional radiology have created less invasive procedures that sometimes mean less surgical pain—and therefore less complicated anesthesia with fewer adverse outcomes. We've already seen the radiological treatment of intracranial aneurysms and arteriovenous malformations, described in chapter 8, which have eliminated the need to open up the skull. Hopefully, the future will see a diminished need for open-heart surgery, as coronary arteries are cleared and valves replaced by thoracoscopy (endoscopic procedures in the chest). Perhaps the interventional radiologists of the twenty-first century will be using lasers to remove plaque from arteries and calcifications from heart valves.

Alternative Forms of Pain Relief

Acupuncture, as I noted in chapter 16, has enjoyed considerable success in certain cultures. When I visited China during the 1970s, I saw a craniotomy (operation in which the skull is opened) being performed under acupuncture anesthesia. The acupuncture was only partially effective, since Demerol was also being administered intravenously, but it did provide a significant level of pain relief. If the reasons for acupuncture's effectiveness in these cultures can be identified, this understanding might lead to even simpler techniques for stimulating endorphin production. We could then place needles in certain areas to produce significant amounts of these naturally occurring narcotics during surgery, making the administration of anesthesia far less complicated.

In the same way, discovering the mechanisms behind the effectiveness of hypnosis and biofeedback may lead us to other less complex forms of pain relief. An intriguing possibility is suggested by studies which found that certain frequencies of music can increase pain thresholds, possibly reducing the need for anesthesia. Once such mechanisms are understood and sharply focused for maximum effect, music as well as the other alternative modalities may become forms of complication-free anesthesia of the future.

A final alternative possibility lies in herbs. In chapter 5 I described the potential adverse effects of common herbal remedies. But we look forward to identifying other herbs with pain-relieving capabilities that lack the serious side effects of the coca plant and the opium poppy.

Tomorrow's Critical Care Medicine

With patients treated increasingly as outpatients, and surgery performed more and more in surgeons' offices, the hospital of the future, I believe, will turn into a large intensive care unit. At the same time, the high cost of caring for these critically ill patients will need to be offset by advances in technology. One possibility is development of computerized feedback systems incorporating microdialysis, a technique that inserts small catheters into various parts of the body to measure for hormones or other parameters and then administers drugs or other substances necessary to correct whatever imbalances are found. For example, an electrode or microchip placed in an artery could continuously and accurately measure oxygen and send this information to a respirator that increases or decreases the oxygen level as needed.

We might even be able to do this monitoring noninvasively. A total body scanner using infrared radiation (much like a pulse oximeter), which could detect substances such as glucose and oxygen in the blood, would be connected to feedback loops, which in turn would be connected to a centralized monitoring system for observation. Fewer staff would be needed; their job would be to reprogram these computers, which would be actually managing the patients.

Less Invasive Pain Management

Although our progress in chronic pain management has been rapid, as I explained in chapter 16, the future will see still better, less invasive ways to manage complex pain syndromes. Again, understanding specific neural transmission routes for pain perception will enable us to develop new ways to interrupt pain signals. For example, researchers are now talking about placing a microchip into a nerve fiber next to the painful area. The chip would receive signals from an external device activated by the patient when pain occurs.

Another innovation would use pellets containing different narcotics or other drugs, inserted around the spinal cord by means of intrathecal catheters. Sustained release of drugs from the pellets could relieve pain over a six-month period.

Finally, preventing pain transmission by electrical stimulation will be simpler in the future, as we become able to direct laser-focused electrical currents to the nerves in question. A small stimulator unit containing the laser could be taped onto the low back, then activated by the patient with a remote device, much like a garage door opener.

As I look back on the state of anesthesia twenty-five years ago, as reflected in Sally's story, it seems we've come pretty far in a relatively short period of time. Yet with the increasing capabilities that modern medical and computer technology has given us, progress should speed up still more. Within the next ten years, many of the applications I've described here as speculation will become reality—and anesthesia will less and less resemble being "put to sleep."

Afterword

· · ·

My hope is that this book leaves you with a sense of patient activism—that it's given you a vocabulary and a road map that will help you make medical decisions, not just about anesthesia but about whatever medical challenges you may be facing. I've included many stories here to help you remember that we physicians are human. Some of us trained many years ago, and, in any case, in today's world of managed care, we find ourselves too rushed to remember everything we should remember. We must see many patients, and sometimes we forget you, your symptoms, and your needs. For this reason, you must help us maximize your chances for well being and even survival.

With the information this book provides, you have the opportunity to become part of a medical team to manage the care of your family, your friends, and even yourself. You need no longer rely on implicit trust that your physician will provide optimal care, for you have the information you need to ask the important questions. Besides, you know now that total trust is just not possible: the doctor has bad days, may lack up-to-date knowledge as a result of being trained years ago, may be hurried and forgetful, or may have his own problems on his mind.

Remember that doctors practicing today were chosen for admission to medical schools based on their performance in the sciences. For years, I believe, this criterion has tended to produce physicians who were weak on the caring side of medical care. Recently, medical school admissions committees have begun looking more for applicants who have volunteered with community groups, senior citizens, or people with AIDS, and have been involved in extracurricular activities in the arts. The committees also now closely examine the applicant's reasons for going into medicine, and those who indicate a strong interest in caring for patients receive preference over those with only a scientific interest in medical research. In the future, I hope, the stereotype of the cold, indifferent doctor, interested only in numbers from laboratory tests, will no longer represent a true picture.

If the future does bring us too many physicians, as many studies have indicated will happen, that may eliminate some of the problems this book has described by making those physicians more available to spend time with you. And if a fortunate circumstance brings everyone in this country basic health insurance, HMOs will no longer be preventing people from getting the care they need, or limiting their anesthetic choices or their time with their doctors.

In the meantime, though, you must know how to take care of yourself. Besides, even under the best health care system imaginable, it's always good to be proactive in an area of life so crucial to your very survival.

Glossary of Common Anesthetic Drugs

• • •

Sedatives

Etomidate, used to induce loss of consciousness, though less often than thiopental. May be preferable for people subject to low blood pressure since it does not depress the heart.

Midazolam, used infrequently to induce loss of consciousness. It has significant amnestic effects and may be used to ensure that a patient won't remember the surgery, Since it does not depress the heart, it is also indicated for patients who may be subject to low blood pressure,

Propofol, commonly used to induce loss of consciousness, especially for ambulatory surgery, since it is shorter acting than thiopental. It also decreases the likelihood of nausea and vomiting.

Thiopental, the drug most commonly used to induce loss of consciousness; short acting.

Inhalation Anesthetics

Desflurane, has a potency similar to isoflurane, but a shorter duration of action; infrequently used.

Halothane, potent, longer-acting than isoflurane, used only for pediatric patients having long procedures,

Isoflurane, potent, used for long procedures.

Nitrous oxide, the most commonly used inhalation anesthetic for maintaining analgesia and amnesia.

Sevoflurane, potency similar to isoflurane and desflurane, but has the shortest duration of action; useful for ambulatory procedures and to induce anesthesia in children.

Muscle Relaxants

Atracurium, same as cisatracurium, but with a somewhat longer duration of action.

Cisatracurium, short-acting, useful for ambulatory procedures.

Pancuronium, longer-acting, used to maintain muscle relaxation during longer procedures.

Rocuronium, same as pancuronium, but somewhat shorter acting.

Succinylcholine, very short-acting, used primarily for patients with potentially difficult airways.

Local Anesthetics

Bupivacaine, commonly used for spinal and epidural anesthesia; longer duration of action than lidocaine. It is also often infused via implantable pumps to treat chronic pain.

Lidocaine, the local anesthetic most often used for regional blocks, with an intermediate duration of action.

Mepivacaine, commonly used for regional blocks, with a shorter duration of action than lidocaine.

Procaine, shortest-acting local anesthetic; commonly used for brief procedures, particularly in the mouth.

Ropivacaine, similar in potency and duration of action to bupivacaine, but less likely to cause cardiac arrest.

Narcotics

Codeine, given orally after surgery to treat mild pain.

Fentanyl, potent synthetic narcotic used to provide analgesia during most operations.

Hydroxycodone, stronger than codeine, used to treat more severe postoperative pain.

Meperidine (Demerol), synthetic narcotic mostly given intramuscularly for postoperative pain management.

Morphine, potent naturally occurring narcotic, commonly given intravenously and intramuscularly to control chronic pain and for patient-controlled anesthesia.

Remifentanyl, potent, shortest-acting synthetic narcotic; usually given as a continuous infusion during surgery.

Sufentanyl, potent synthetic narcotic, shorter acting than fentanyl and longer acting than remifentanyl.

Index

• • •

About the Authors

. . .

James E. Cottrell, M.D., is first vice-president for scientific affairs of the American Society of Anesthesiologists and chairman and professor of the department of anesthesiology at SUNY Health Science Center at Brooklyn, where he is also senior associate dean for clinical practice and past president of the medical staff.

He is the coeditor of *Anesthesia and Neurosurgery* (Mosby, 1994) and *Neuroanesthesia: Handbook of Clinical and Physiologic Essentials* (Little, Brown, 1999) and the author of more than one hundred articles in medical journals, including the *New England Journal of Medicine* and the *Lancet*. He is editor-in-chief of the *Journal of Neurosurgical Anesthesiology* and was a columnist for *Surgical Rounds*.

Cottrell has frequently served as a consultant to and has participated on grants from the National Institutes of Health. He was a health policy adviser to Senator Edward M. Kennedy and the Senate Committee on Labor and Human Resources.

A founding member and chairman of the AIDS Action Foundation, Cottrell currently serves on the honorary board of God's Love We Deliver, an organization in Manhattan that daily feeds approximately eight hundred homebound people with AIDS. He is a member of the board of Doctors of the World.

Stephanie Golden is a medical writer and award-winning nonfiction author whose books include *The Women Outside: Meanings and Myths of Homelessness* and *Slaying the Mermaid: Women and the Culture of Sacrifice.*